Kareen Zebroff, happily married mother of three, bestselling author of four books, lecturer-demonstrator, researcher, Yoga and Nutrition expert, organic gardener and health food cook, qualified school teacher, sparkles with good health and *joie de vivre*. For the seven short years since she first took up Yoga she has changed from tense and brittle to graceful and flexible. Good nutrition practices and the soothing Yoga poses have transformed an overweight housewife with debilitating symptoms of anxiety, irritability and lack of energy, into a relaxed and joyous person. Now she shares her secret with you . . .

The ABC of Yoga

Kareen Zebroff

CORGI BOOKS
A DIVISION OF TRANSWORLD PUBLISHERS LTD

THE ABC OF YOGA

A CORGI BOOK   0 552 98057 9

First publication in Great Britain

PRINTING HISTORY

Corgi edition published 1978

Copyright © Fforbez Enterprises Ltd. 1971

Photographs by Duncan McDougall, Vancouver, B.C.

Edited by Kenneth D. McRae

Corgi Books are published by Transworld Publishers Ltd.,
Century House, 61–63 Uxbridge Road, Ealing, London, W5 5SA

Made and printed in Great Britain by
Richard Clay (The Chaucer Press), Ltd., Bungay, Suffolk.

To my Mother
who started me
on the
Royal Path
of
Yoga

INTRODUCTION

WHY THIS BOOK WAS WRITTEN

After a few months' airing of my T.V. show it became obvious that I should have to write a book. By that time I had received over 2,000 letters requesting information about books and exercises and about how to apply Yoga to the individual's need. Many viewers wrote to say that they did not have the time nor inclination to wade through pages of a philosophical treatise or gushy generalities. They did not want to be sold; all they wanted was a "how-to" sort of book that stated precisely and concisely how to do the various Yoga postures and what their benefits were.

That is exactly what I have attempted to do here. Having, myself, first become acquainted with Yoga through a book, I know exactly what I want to find in such a book and what I could well do without. Here it is easy to find the postures because they are alphabetically arranged; the benefits are stated first, because most people want to know what they will get from their efforts before they start them; the exercises follow an explicit, step-by-step plan to make easier the glancing back at the page for further instruction as one little by little, gets into a position; dos and don'ts guide you in avoiding the most common errors; an exercise schedule plan in the back of the book will suit every individual's need or capacity; and finally, for specific health or appearance worries, a list of exercises suggests an appropriate Yoga exercise to help you overcome your problem.

A purist might easily object here to the westernized version of the Yoga I am describing in this book. But since we *are* Westerners with an entirely different life-style, life-attitude, life-pace and even physical tradition (we do not squat or sit cross-legged from the time we are toddlers) from the original Yogis of the East, such an objection is merely academic. What the average reader will most be interested in is the question "will it work for me?" My answer to that is an enthusiastic "yes", which has only one condition attached to it: regular practice. Because, whether your problem is tension or weight-control, getting old or lack of energy, sagging muscles or a weak or injured back, sluggish digestive processes or a wrinkled face, you will find that Yoga works for you and works wonders. Can you imagine the sort of letter you would write to your teacher if, after years of futile attempts, your problem suddenly exists no more with the practice of Yoga? That is the sort of grateful testimonial to the art of Yoga I receive daily from my viewers.

I know just what these people are talking about, because three years ago I was twenty pounds overweight and quite depressed. Buried in an isolated northern community with three small children under the age of 5, I was constantly tired. The children seemed to be ill all that year, the company-town was typically clannish and eventually I was full of self-pity. Then my mother wrote, urging me to study Yoga, because she had found it so beneficial to her at a trying time of life.

That is when my life changed. Together with a sensible diet low in carbohydrates, and the Yoga exercises, I dropped the over-weight within 3 months. My energy-level improved one-hundred percent and so did my outlook on life. I became more cheerful and patient with the children, attacked my chores with verve and concentration and looked and felt prettier with improved posture and complexion. My body became firm and streamlined and I lost inches everywhere, particularly in my inherited trouble-spot, the inner thigh. People said I looked years younger. But best of all was my tremendous feeling of vitality, of being ALIVE, of being ME, and liking it. Now, a day that does not include the Headstand, the Shoulderstand and the Abdominal Lift is not complete.

CONTENTS

INFORMATION

WHAT YOGA IS ALL ABOUT

Most people are now familiar with the word "Yoga". But the exact meaning may be shrouded in visions of bearded sages lying on beds of nails or standing on their heads at the oddest times. That may be an extreme form of Yoga practiced by fanatics but it has nothing to do with the proper study of Yoga laid out in the Sanskrit text books. Neither is Yoga the way-out prerogative of the young.

More and more young people are, of course, discovering meditation as an alternative to going on a trip with the aid of drugs. But the beauty of Yoga lies in its great versatility, which can please and benefit anyone of any age, creed or sex. It is one of the few things in life where results are almost immediate. What then is it and what can it do?

Basically, there are two broad areas of Yoga: Hatha Yoga, consisting of the asanas or exercises, and Meditative Yoga, of which there exist five main forms. For instance, there is Jnana Yoga, a meditative technique (through knowledge) for the intellectual. A muscial person might choose Mantra Yoga in which a trance-like state is achieved through repetitious chanting. A Salvation Army officer is actually practising a form of Bhakti Yoga, which is the Yoga of love and service.

However, Hatha Yoga, with which we are concerned here, is the only physical discipline among the lot. True, it is only a small part of the whole but it is a most important part, because it represents the first step on the ladder to the ultimate goal of samadhi, or self-realization. It disciplines the body, so that the mind is free to expand. The *Yoga Sara Sangraha*, defines Yoga as: "the silencing of the mind's activities through physical and mental self-discipline which leads to the complete realization of the intrinsic nature of the "Supreme Person". The "Supreme Person" may be thought of as the ultimate best in all of us, the image of God in our hearts. Yoga, meaning yoke or union, shows us the path, and no matter what your religion, Yoga will enhance it for you.

In order to have the mind free, one must first be able to forget the body. That is only possible if everything is in perfect running order, if no aches and pains distract from meditation. Just as one cannot possibly enjoy the beauties of nature gliding by if the automobile in which one is sitting has developed a mysterious knock, or broken springs, so it is impossible to sit for any period in concentrated thought if a throbbing pain is to be felt in stiff muscles or if one's back is aching. Hatha Yoga is concerned with organic health, not the physical development of the muscles, although that is a very pleasant and certain side-effect.

The "art" of Yoga itself is 5,000 years old, and it was first put into written form 2,500 years ago. Hatha Yoga comprises breathing techniques, rituals of hygiene and physical exercises. The latter were refined from the observation of the stretching movements of jungle animals. After all, who is more lithe, relaxed and healthy than the cat family? What does a cat do immediately upon getting up or lying down? Stretch. STRETCHING is tranquilizing. Hatha Yoga is the best physical culture system in the world. It relaxes, rejuvenates, tones, firms, regulates body-functions, energizes and beautifies. Through regular, half-hour practices you can drastically change your life.

For instance, were you aware that right now, sitting there improperly in your chair, you are only using 1/5th of your total lung-power? Can you imagine how much more energetic, vital and healthy you would feel with just 10 minutes of proper daily deep-breathing? If you are yawning right now, you are probably sitting in a stuffy room, the carbon-dioxide level in your blood stream has exceeded a safety-level and your yawn is an immediate demand of your body for OXYGEN NOW! As for diet, there is an isolated tribe living in the mountains near Pakistan whose members are incredibly long-lived and astoundingly disease-free. Why? Their diet is very low on carbohydrates. So it is in Yoga.

The secret lies in stretching muscles, not tensing them as you do in calisthenics; in moving slowly, so that one can stop immediately the warning-signal of pain appears. It is to be found in Personal Progress, in which you compare yourself to no-one else, only to yourself as you were yesterday, so that no matter what your age, flexibility or state of health, you can exercise safely and with success. You go as far as *you* can and hold it there until you're uncomfortable. By this action you are exercising over and over as it were, and therefore have to do an exercise only 2 or 3 times instead of 20. This loosens and strengthens the muscles in preparation for your ultimate goal.

Yoga renews energy where calisthenics deplete it. It relieves you of minor aches and pains, of constipation and of hemorrhoids. If your abdominal wall is in a pitiable state after several child-births, if you have arthritis, bursitis, sciatica, or disc-problems, Yoga can supply some helpful exercises. If your legs ache at the end of the day, if you suffer from insomnia or can't unwind even in sleep, if you are irritable or uncomfortable, Yoga can help you.

WHY YOU SHOULD PRACTICE YOGA

Yoga is primarily concerned with organic health. It is a system of exercising devised to keep you healthy for as long as you live and thereby to increase your life-span. There must be no gradual decline in the efficiency of body-functions or body mechanisms as you advance in age. The animal in its natural habitat does not develop a general debility. It either dies violently or retains its ability to care for its body until it dies at the age normal for its species.

Maintaining one's health throughout a normal age-span brings with it many benefits, such as a youthful bearing and outlook, a feeling of energy, beauty, poise, and the ability to relax.

Of these, YOUTH, or in the case of an elderly person, REJUVEN-ATION is the most important. If your spine is limber and flexible at 55, then for all intents and purposes you are a supple 30. If, however, your back is stiff and tense at 20, your age could logically be put at 60. You are as old as your spine; keep it young and flexible and you will be young and flexible too.

The spinal column is an amazing piece of machinery. It is extremely flexible, being able to bend forward, backward, sideways and even spirally. This is made possible because the spine consists of separate pieces of bone which are kept from grinding on each other by little parts or discs. The primary function of the spine is to provide housing for that most important extension of the brain: the central and autonomic nervous system, consisting of the spinal cord. From this, nerves extend to every part of the body, so that the brain is always in close contact with all of it. The importance of keeping the spinal column healthy and flexible is self-evident.

However, the spine is only a part of the whole. No part of the body is entirely separate from the next. Everything that takes place causes a chain-reaction. For instance, under mental or physical tension, you are contracting muscles which are unable to work at full capacity. This contraction, in turn, inactivates the tendons and ligaments; the joints are not being "oiled", and become stiff. As a result, you become physically uncomfortable, irritable, devoid of energy, sick, depressed and more tense: the vicious cycle is complete.

Another important factor in maintaining health and thereby beauty, is often overlooked: circulation. According to the theory of evolution, we started out as a species, on all-fours. In this position, the heart lies under the spinal column and most of the body is in a horizontal stance -- all of which makes it easier for the circulatory system to keep every part of the body supplied with rich blood. In an upright stance we sacrifice many of the conditions for perfect health. Because of gravitational pull, the head gets very little circulation and one suffers accordingly from a lack of alertness and a sallow complexion. Abdominal organs lose their elasticity over the years, sag and exert pressure on each other, pushing out the abdominal wall. This condition in turn cuts off badly-needed circulation in the pelvic area where important hormone-producing glands (=YOUTH) are located. It also puts a great strain on the intercostal muscles which are attached to the skeleton. The result — abdominal, back, sexual and other health problems. Of course, the legs are affected also and fatigue, varicose veins, tension, and other unpleasant conditions result. No wonder that in Yoga the inverted postures such as the Headstand and the Shoulderstand are considered to be beneficial for any health problem one might name. And, an exercise such as the Abdominal Lift is a must for achieving and maintaining organic health, because it lifts back into place and vigorously massages and stimulates most abdominal organs. Calisthenics is mostly concerned with muscular health, Yoga with organic well-being. The former depletes energy, where the latter renews it.

MEDITATION

A far greater part of Yoga is taken up by meditation than by the physical exercise program of Hatha Yoga. However, the latter is a very important and necessary step up the ladder of self-realization. A person interested in Yoga, as a whole, is most concerned with communing with a higher consciousness, with self-knowledge, or ultimately, with Peace of Mind. There are several paths to this goal. As explained in "WHAT YOGA IS ALL ABOUT" at the beginning of the book, there are enough different meditative techniques to suit each temperament. The meditational Yoga most closely associated with Hatha Yoga, however, is Raja Yoga, or the "Royal Path to Self-Realization".

Yoga aims at a controlling of the mind to where its activities and movements are stilled, so that there may be no distraction from a complete awareness of and contact with the Supreme Person within yourself. Just as you cannot see through a windowpane when pouring rain beats against it, it is impossible to find deep within yourself an image of universal consciousness, if thought obscures it. As the rain slackens and finally stops, you are able to look through the shiny glass at the glorious colours of a rainbow. With patient practice, that is what you can achieve with Yoga. The rainbow can be regarded as a Higher Consciousness, the Supreme Person, the Absolute, or God; the raindrops are your thoughts. The rewards of such thought control are peace of mind, a youthful outlook and denial of the ego, all of which makes you a better person.

In this book there is no place for the description of a meditational technique, but I can give you an idea of the general workings of meditation. Mainly, it follows these steps:

1. A comfortable but upright posture which one can assume for a length of time without movement, usually the Lotus position, in a quiet place.

2. A turning inward of one's senses and thoughts, so that no distraction from the outer world is experienced.

3. A concentration upon an object, such as a candle, an apple, a beautiful picture, until one can see the object in the mind's eye with eyes closed.

4. A contemplation of the object to the exclusion of everything else. This last step is a kind of passive sitting back and watching the thoughts go by, until one is beyond thought.

5. Meditation. It can only be described as an exultation, a moment of intense happiness, a great joy. Most of us have had a momentary contact with meditation, without realizing it. It may have occurred on listening to a piece of music. Or one may have found oneself profoundly stirred by looking at a picture. Sexual love sometimes produces such a moment.

The conditions of meditation are essentially met by following the Ten Commandments. It is not only necessary to commit no immoral acts but also to harbor no negative feelings or emotions, such as fear, anger, jealousy. And even if one does not come to it pure, meditation will help one to achieve the goal. Raja Yoga cleans house in one's mind and thereby strengthens it, makes it more alert and active; Hatha Yoga teaches control over body; the two of them are a powerfully good combination.

DIET

To put it very simply, the daily Yoga diet could be described as a natural one. This means that all foods are eaten as close to their natural state as possible. Flour should not be refined or bleached, but whole wheat; sugar should be raw or in the form of honey, or not eaten at all (since a normal day's fare of proteins, fruits, vegetables and grains contains the equivalent of 2 cups of sugar); vegetables should be steamed or baked to a soft crispness only or preferably eaten raw; rice should be unpolished (brown), noodles and all baked foods should be made from whole wheat; nuts and dried fruits should be an important part of the diet and so should yogurt; fruits and vegetables should be organically grown, without the use of insecticides, herbicides and chemical fertilizers. Rule of thumb: if it is white and refined, if it is instant, if it has chemical additives in it, if it has been chemically changed (hydrogenation of fats) — it's a no-no.

The Yogi considers the body as the temple of his soul. As such he has the responsibility to keep it from falling into ruin. However, it only houses the spirit and as such, a stomach-consciousness must be avoided. The Yogi eats a little several times a day, but only when he is hungry. He chews thoroughly, eats slowly, knowing that digestion starts in the mouth, where enzymes contained in the saliva provide the first of several breaking-up processes. Such small meals might consist of a handful of sprouted seeds, or a little bowl of yogurt. It might be a bite of cheese, a banana or some dried fruits and nuts. But never is his meal huge. He knows moderation in all things. He will be aware of the need to get sufficient protein in his diet, since he very often is a vegetarian. He knows that seeds, such as sunflowerseeds, soybeans, wheatgerm, brewer's yeast and nuts are an excellent source of complete protein. So are, as combinations, legumes and grains, beans or nuts and milk, and brown rice and sesame seeds. Dairy products, of course, all have the eight essential amino acids, which are needed to make up a complete protein. Nor are these foods necessarily fattening. It is entirely possible to lose weight on a diet of beans and milk. However, a balanced diet is what the Yogi believes in, with plenty of fresh fruits and vegetables.

But what of a losing diet? Of all the fad diets now so popular on the market, it can be said after considerable research, that the low-calorie diet in conjunction with vitamin supplements that help to metabolize the food and acts as natural diuretics, is still the most lasting and the healthiest. To change one's eating habits, to develop a mind consciousness, is the key. The calorie is not a food, but solely a unit of measurement. You need X number of calories in order to produce Y amount of heat. The more heat you use by exerting yourself physically, the more calories are burned. This is why a former football player will suddenly go to fat after he enters business, even though he doesn't eat more. He simply exercises less. There is a definite correlation between exercise and diet:

1. exercise + diet = maximum weight loss
2. exercise without diet = maintaining weight
3. no exercise and diet = maintaining weight
4. no exercise and no diet = weight gain

Since refined foods consist of "empty" calories — they have no nutritive values such as protein, vitamins, minerals and fatty acids — you can remove them from your diet forever. Did you know that sugar is addictive? If you wean yourself gradually from sugar and white flour products, you will not only feel a great surge in energy, and experience a most satisfying weight loss, but you will soon find all candies and cakes and ice cream sickeningly sweet.

HOW TO PRACTICE YOGA

Different people hope to achieve different benefits through the practice of Yoga. The teenager is primarily concerned about spot-improving a not-quite-perfect figure. The typical housewife with several small children will want to increase her energy and lose a few flabby pounds. A middle-aged person needs to rid himself of several years' mounted-up tension and bad habits, be they eating, drinking or smoking; and the elderly have become aware of aches, pains and stiffness. They know something must be done to get the spring back into their step and to enjoy again the taste of food and the resting qualities of deep sleep. Put all those needs together and they spell H-E-A-L-T-H. But, they also spell W-O-R-K. However, the nice thing about Yoga is that it does add up to a lot of expended effort, but doesn't feel like it. It gets tremendous results, but does not exhaust you. Even after a knee-shaking Yoga work-out, you will not suffer from muscular soreness if you follow the sensible rules laid out here. For maximum benefit with a minimum of effort, please consider all these points every time you practise Yoga.

Time

The best time to exercise is either first thing in the morning or last thing at night. It depends on your particular need. In the morning the body is still stiff, but the exercises will help you to work better all day. In the evening the exercising comes more easily and refreshes and relaxes you for a good sleep.

Place

A private, airy place where you can expect little interruption is best. For, the more you concentrate, the better you will do each exercise. A rug or a blanket folded in four will give you good protection from the hard floor without being too soft for efficient performance.

Food

It is wise not to exercise strenuously for at least two hours after a heavy meal and one hour after a light meal, but it is permissible to take a little liquid just before.

Hygiene

The Yoga postures are done more easily after a bath, especially if you are a tense or arthritic person. Always empty the bladder and move the bowels before the practice of Yoga. You will find that constipation is no longer a problem with regular practice, but since the upside-down poses promote elimination, it is advisable to start your program with these.

For The Ladies

You may exercise during menstruation if you wish - on a lighter scale than normal, however. But do not ever practise the inverted postures such as the Shoulderstand. It is quite safe to practise Yoga during pregnancy for the first three months, or longer, but you should always check with your doctor first. There are special exercises to make the muscles of the back strong and elastic, to strengthen the floor of the pelvis, and to master deep breathing techniques as aids to labour.

High Blood Pressure, Dizziness or Detached Retina

People who suffer from any of these complaints should always check with their doctor. They should not at first do any of the inverted postures such as the Shoulderstand, but any of the forward bending poses are beneficial. To experience a certain amount of dizziness in the beginning is quite normal, since the head usually gets little circulation. In the inverted postures there is a sudden onrush of blood dilating the blood vessels, and a slight headache or dizziness may result.

Yoga Asanas (Postures)

There is no doubt that Yoga can work miracles. But the instrument through which wonders are worked is you. Without your discipline, your faith in what you are doing and your persistence in doing it, there can be no results. There is a right and a wrong way of practising Yoga and often a little variation will make all the difference. Try to come to the practice of Yoga without preconceived notions of how to do the exercise. Read or listen to instructions fully and to the end. Too often people will listen half-way, think they know what is going to be said next, and go ahead and do their own incomplete and/or incorrect effort.

No matter what your age, Yoga can help you realize your secret bodily desire: be it energy, health, beauty, youthfulness or graceful bearing - - if you practise regularly and sensibly.

THE DOS AND DON'TS OF
PRACTISING YOGA ASANAS

1. *Practise regularly*, even if you have time for only a few exercises on some days. Then, do only those that you know do *you* the most good. If you suffer from tension, do the Chest Expander; if your tummy is flabby, concentrate on the Pump, and so on. But make Yoga as much of your daily routine as eating and sleeping. The change in your health and outlook on life will make it worthwhile a hundred times over.

2. *Never hurry*. Go into the postures *slowly*, taking 10 - 15 seconds to get from the beginning to the holding position. This gives bonus benefits and makes each exercise more effective. It also helps to cut down on the number of times an exercise has to be done.

3. *Hold each posture* once you have gone as far into it as comfort permits. Muscles must receive sustained strain in order to stay in condition. As a beginner, hold each posture at its extremity for 5 seconds. Increase this time by 5 seconds a week as you improve. Through the holding position you are doing an exercise over and over as it were, and therefore an exercise need be done only three times, instead of twenty.

4. *Come out of an exercise* as *slowly* as you went into it. You lose at least a third of the value if you permit yourself to collapse, and you might even risk injury.

5. *Never force a position*, never jerk or bounce in order to "go further". Go as far as you can, then hold it there. Pain is a danger-signal devised by the body to stop immediately or risk injury. If, as in calisthenics, you are moving so fast that your momentum does not permit you to stop short, you can easily move past the danger-signal and get hurt. This is what happens when you experience muscular soreness or muscle-strain.

6. *Never compare yourself to anyone else.* Yoga emphasizes "Personal Progress". By performing the exercise regularly you are bound to do better today than you did yesterday. In going to the limit of your capability you receive the same benefits as your teacher who can stretch much further but who is also more flexible. In Yoga there is visible progress. You will find that after a time you can get into poses you would never have dreamed possible.

7. *Concentrate fiercely* with each exercise you perform. It will follow naturally that you then do the exercise well. This is especially necessary in balancing exercises. Moving your head rapidly, or speaking or laughing embarrassedly when you do lose your balance will retard your progress and efficiency. Simply carry on where you left off without a feeling of disgust or embarrassment at yourself. Then your concentration will remain unbroken and you can achieve much. Visualizing encourages concentration which in turn promotes quality of action. For instance, pretend to be a fierce lion in the Lion or a pussy-cat just up from her nap in the Cat Stretch. It will make exercising more fun for you too.

8. *Rest between exercises.* The beauty of Yoga lies in its gentleness. You need never experience draining fatigue or painful, sore muscles. Catch your breath, let the muscles rebound from a delightful stretch and permit the body to assimilate what it has learned.

9. *Breathe normally* during the holding position of an exercise. There is a tendency for most people to hold their breath while they desperately and tensely hold on. This is absolutely wrong. Yoga stresses relaxation, even while exercising. If at all possible, you should go as far into a pose as comfort permits, then relax there and breathe normally. As a student advances in proficiency there is a prescribed way of breathing with each exercise. For the beginner, it suffices to become thoroughly familiar with the performing technique of the Yoga postures, before learning the breathing technique.

BREATH CONTROL

Hatha Yoga is made up of three main parts: exercise, acts of body-cleansing, and breath-control. Of these, the Yogis consider the last of highest priority, because air is our most important food for both body and mind. In the Sanskrit language of the ancient Yogis, breath control is called PRANA-YAMA. Prana means "breath" or more accurately, "life-force", and ayama means "pause" or "control". The Yogis believe in an invisible cosmic force around us, the mysterious essence which gives us life, a kind of universal energy. Without prana you are dead; the more you have of it, the more alive and energetic you are. By mastering proper breathing techniques, you increase your "living" potential. You can become more alert and aware -- master of yourself.

If you were to conduct a scientific experiment with yourself, you would discover that you can do without solids for over a month; you can survive without liquids or sleep for about a week, but without oxygen you would perish within minutes. However, if you attempted to hold your breath indefinitely (as small children will attempt to do as a means to getting their way) you would merely *become unconscious* and then an automatic breathing control would take over involuntarily. However, in view of its importance, it is amazing how much *conscious* control also we have over our breathing. Without that we could not express our emotions through laughing, sobbing, exulting or sighing. How much breathing influences our emotions is evident through simple observation. If you are excited or nervous you will breathe more rapidly than when quietly resting. And vice-versa, you can always "take a tranquilizer" of several deep breaths to calm yourself or your nervous system. For instance, thousands of insomniacs have found the Alternate Nostril Breath particularly beneficial. Regulating your breathing calms the mind, refreshes the spirit, prolongs life by slowing down the heartbeat, aids the digestion, and purifies the bloodstream which improves the complexion and increases energy.

In order to understand how this is possible one must have an elementary understanding of the breathing-process. Oxygen serves two main functions in the body. First, every single cell of the several billion in the body has to breathe by receiving cell-repairing oxygen and discharging the waste matter called carbon-dioxide. Second, oxygen is needed to change food into energy. It "fans the fires of combustion", so to speak. The more energetic you are, the more oxygen you need.

Ordinarily, the body can get 1/2 pint of oxygen from breathing in 5 quarts of air a minute. An athlete will need as many as 100 quarts or more. The lung, normally, can hold 5 - 6 quarts of air at a time. Since you are, as of this minute, using only 1/5 of your total lung power, you will realize how poorly you are using your natural resources.

Obviously, it is necessary to re-learn how to breathe properly. Technically speaking, the following happens. Your lungs contract and expand like a bellows up to twenty times a minute. The muscle controlling this action is the diaphragm. It is dome-shaped and inflates the lungs by flattening out, thereby pulling on the intercostal muscles. These, in turn, pull apart the rib-cage and the air is now permitted to flood into the bottom of the pear-shaped lungs. To make the diaphragm flatten out, one must push the abdomen out, which is exactly the opposite of what most of us do when inhaling. To breathe properly is especially difficult for women, who have been told all their lives to "push the chest out and pull the tummy in", and who have worn tight girdles, belts and corsets for many years.

Technically speaking, there are certain steps to proper breathing which must be observed in all breathing exercises:

1. All breathing must be done through the nose, which acts as a filter and prevents the lungs from clogging. As air travels through the nose it is warmed, moistened and cleaned of impurities. A famous Yogi once said, "the mouth is for eating and kissing, the nose for breathing".

2. You should always sit in a straight-backed position to straighten out the thorax. For the asthma-sufferer the Fish asana is prescribed, which throws the head far back to facilitate breathing.

3. Breathe outdoors whenever possible, or in front of an open window.

4. You should deep-breathe for about 10 minutes a day to receive the maximum benefits: an energetic body, a tranquil mind and a serene emotional outlook.

5. For a "hold" position it is recommended to use a chin-lock. This is done by lowering your head and resting it tightly against the jugular notch between the collar bones. When the holding period is over, usually after 5 seconds, raise your head again for the exhalation.

6. Attempt to breathe noiselessly, except in the Cleansing Breath and Cooling Breath where a hissing sound should be heard.

7. Breathe and perform the body-movements involved rhythmically, smoothly and slowly for greatest benefit.

8. On an inhalation, concentrate on expanding the ribs and pushing the abdomen out.

9. On an exhalation always tuck the abdomen in as far as it will go, to expel all old and stale air.

YOGA

EXERCISES

(ASANAS)

46 EXERCISES FOR BETTER HEALTH

ABDOMINAL LIFT

I. *Benefits:*

The Abdominal Lift ——
- strengthens and firms the *abdominal muscles.*
- reduces the *waistline.*
- promotes *regularity* and relieves *constipation* by stimulating the peristaltic action of the *colon.*
- tones and massages most *abdominal organs* and *glands.*
- improves circulation to the abdominal area which aids the *digestion* and *metabolism.*

II. *Technique:*

1. Stand straight, the legs about a foot apart.
2. Bend forwards placing your hands just above the knees and shifting your weight onto them.
3. Inhale and then EXHALE FULLY and do not breathe again throughout the exercise. It is of the greatest importance that no breath should be left in the body.
4. Relax the abdomen and pull it inward and then upward as though to have the navel touch the spine. This creates a deep hollow. (Figure 1)
5. Hold the inward pull for one second and then bang the abdomen out in a sudden motion.
6. Immediately pull the abdomen in again, remembering to also give the upward pull which should be so strong that it tightens the muscles of the neck. (Figure 2)
7. Bang the abdomen out again after one second, etc.
8. Repeat this in and out motion for a total of 3-5 times on the one exhalation.
9. Relax, gasping for air. If you find that you are exhaling as you straighten out, you will have done the exercise wrong.
10. Perform a set of 3-5 contractions each three times and if you are really concerned about constipation or slack muscles, then do this three times a day.

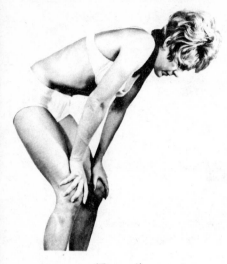

(Figure 1)

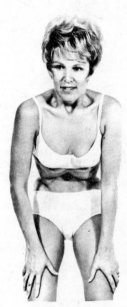

(Figure 2)

III. *Dos and Don'ts:*

DO make sure that your lungs are completely empty before pulling the
abdomen in. This will take a little practice and you may find that
you tend to breathe in with each inward pull. The 3-5 contractions
are all performed on one breath.

DO have your abdomen relaxed to permit a proper hollowing.

DO work up your contractions to 10 on one exhalation as you advance,
but do it gradually at one extra contraction a week.

DON'T get discouraged if your abdomen is fat and doesn't seem to hollow at all. That emaciated look will just take a little longer to
achieve, but it will happen.

ALTERNATE LEG STRETCH

I.   *Benefits:*

The Alternate Leg Stretch ——
- strengthens and firms the *abdomen* and *legs.*
- reduces *tension* from the *legs, buttocks* and *back.*
- massages most *abdominal organs* and stimulates them into action.
- *rejuvenates* by making the *spine* supple and strong.

II.   *Technique:*

1. Sit on the floor, legs stretched out, back straight.
2. Bend your left leg and, keeping the side of the knee on the floor, bring your left foot against the right thigh, close to the body. (Figure 3)
3. Stretching the arms out, slide them SLOWLY down your leg as far as you can reach, bending forward with a curling motion of the spine. (Figure 4)
4. Grasp the leg; this may be at the knee, calf or ankle, depending on your flexibility.
5. Bend the elbows out and down, and gently pull yourself forward and down. Avoid strain by making this a smooth, not jerky, motion.
6. Go only as far as you comfortably can and then hold the position 5-30 seconds. Breathe normally. (Figure 5)
7. Straighten up slowly and repeat on the other side.
8. Perform three times on each side.

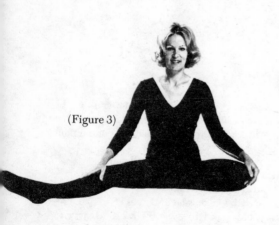

(Figure 3)

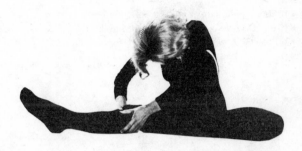

(Figure 4)

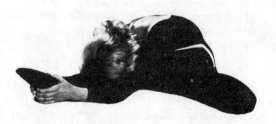

(Figure 5)

III. *Dos and Don'ts:*

It is amazing how quickly, with perseverance, you will be able to bring your head to your knee. A stiff spine and tense hamstring muscles are one of the first indications of age. This asana will loosen both areas in even the most inflexible.

DON'T bend your knees and refrain from jerking. It is the motionless holding of the Yoga positions that does the most effective work and prevents strain.

ANKLE BENDS

I. *Benefits:*

The Ankle Bends ——
- relieve swollen *ankles* and *feet*.
- strengthen weak *ankles,* excellent for *skiing*.
- improve *circulation* and remove *fatigue* in legs.
- make *legs* and *ankles* shapely.

II. *Technique:*

1. Stand straight, feet 2 inches apart.
2. Roll to the right onto the sides of your feet. (You will be resting on the outside of the right foot and on the inside of the left foot.) (Figure 6)
3. Bend your knees forward and to the right, but keep your hips and pelvis to the front.
4. Hold the position for 5 seconds or until you begin to be uncomfortable.
5. Repeat on the other side.
6. Now lift the right foot and pointing it forward, rotate the foot full circle from the ankle, first clockwise, then anti-clockwise. (Figure 7)
7. Repeat with the other foot.
8. Perform whole series twice more.

III. *Dos and Don'ts:*

DOing the exercises regularly will keep a youthful spring in your step, as stiff ankles are one of the first signs of old age.
DON'T swivel your pelvis to the side - you would waste your effort.

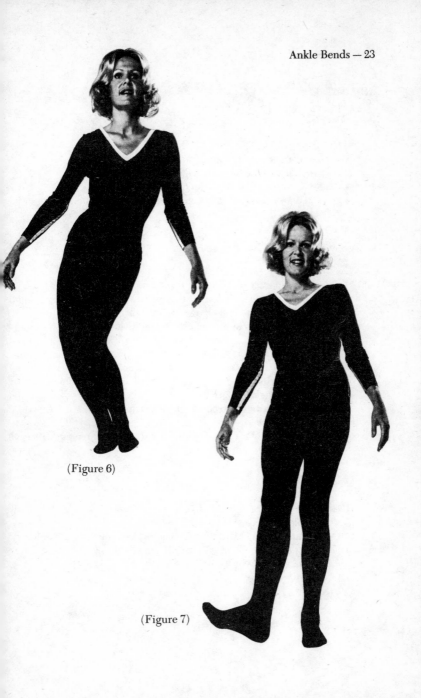

(Figure 6)

(Figure 7)

ARM AND LEG STRETCH

I. *Benefits:*

   The Arm and Leg Stretch —
   - stretches and firms the whole *front of the body*.
   - promotes *grace* and *poise*, through improved balance.
   - relieves *tension* of the *back* and *thighs*.
   - gives a most pleasant massage to *vertebrae* through the gentle *backward stretch*.
   - expands the *chest*.

II. *Technique:*

   1. Stand straight, heels together, toes slightly pointed outward.
   2. Raise your arm slowly so that it stands out at an angle but the hand is above the head. The elbows are straight.
   3. Bend your left leg at the knee, bringing it close to the buttocks, and shift your body weight onto the right foot.
   4. Grasp your left foot with your left hand. (Figure 8)
   5. Bend backward from the waist, at the same time pulling on the foot and moving the right arm as far back as balancing permits. Let the head drop back. (Figure 9)
   6. Hold this position 5 seconds at the start, increasing the time at 5 seconds a week.
   7. Repeat on the other side and perform the asana three times on each side.

III. *Dos and Don'ts:*

   DO simple balancing exercises such as the Tree first, if you have difficulty keeping your balance.
   DO concentrate fiercely, it will help you to keep your balance better.
   DO move slowly when going into and coming out of the Arm and Leg Stretch, as in all Yoga exercises.
   DON'T close your eyes.

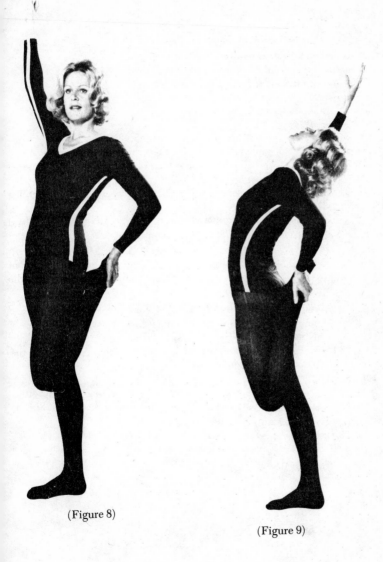

(Figure 8)

(Figure 9)

ARM LIFT

I. *Benefits:*

The Arm Lift ——
- firms flabby *under arms.*
- strengthens and firms the pectoral muscles of the *bustline.*
- relieves *tension* in the *shoulders.*

II. *Technique:*
1. Sit in a comfortably cross-legged position.
2. Bring your hands up to the shoulders, palms up, fingers pointing to the neck and elbows to the side so that the arms form a straight line with the chest. (Figure 10)
3. Slowly raise your hands in the isometric way, resisting the motion all the way up. (Figure 11)
4. Stretch your arms straight and then lower just as slowly, resisting the movement. Breathe normally throughout.
5. Repeat 3-5 times.

III. *Dos and Don'ts:*

DO visualize a great weight to be lifted slowly over your head as it is helpful for best performance. You must lower it just as slowly or it will crush you.

DO push hard, in resistance to the movement, so that the sinews in the arms and fingers stand out.

Rest and breathe normally between each exercise if you wish. Keep in mind that if you have recently lost weight or if you intend to lose it, the baggy look is especially obvious under the arms.

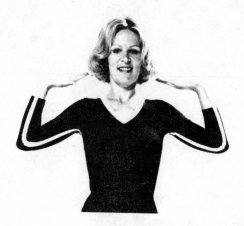

(Figure 10)

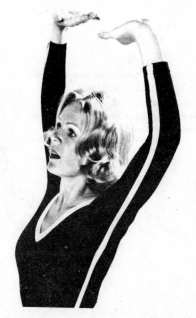

(Figure 11)

BLADE

I. *Benefits*

The Blade ——
- relieves *bursitis* and *arthritic pain*.
- develops and firms pectoral muscles of the *bustline*.
- relieves tension in *shoulders* and *upper back*.

II. *Technique*

1. Sit in a comfortably cross-legged position.
2. Bend your elbows and bring them up at the sides, fingertips touching in front of your chest. (Figure 12)
3. Draw the shoulder blades together as though you had to hold onto a $10 bill between them. Keep elbows up as much as possible.
4. Hold the pose for 5-10 seconds. (Figure 13)
5. Release the pose slowly. Shrug your shoulders.
6. Repeat 3-5 times.

III. *Dos and Donts*

DO relax momentarily tense muscles by shrugging them. The shoulders are usually the first seat of tension and may, at first, complain about being stretched out of their cramped position.

DON'T raise your shoulders as you pinch them and try to keep the elbows up.

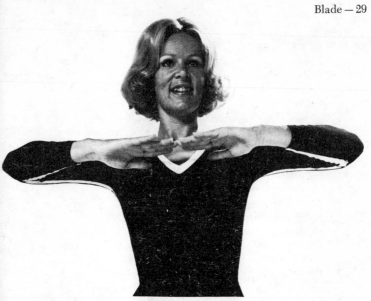

(Figure 12)

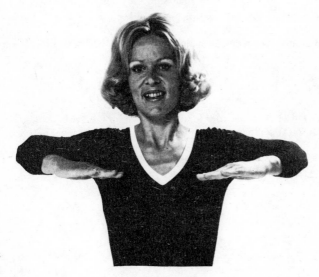

(Figure 13)

BOAT (LOCUST)

I.   *Benefits:*

The Boat ——
- is beneficial to people with a *slipped disc*.
- firms the *buttocks*.
- firms and reduces weight in the *hips*.
- aids *digestion*.
- is beneficial to *bladder* and *sex glands*.
- stretches and limbers up the *spine*.
- relieves pain in the *sacral* and *lumbar areas* of the *back*.
- tightens and flattens the *abdomen*.

II.   *Technique:*

1.   Lie on your stomach on the floor, arms stretched back, face down. (Figure 14)
2.   All at the same time, slowly lift your head, chest and legs as far as they will go.
3.   Lift your arms a few inches off the floor but parallel to it.
4.   Pinch your buttocks together and keep the legs stretched straight and together. (Figure 15)
5.   Hold, breathing normally, for as long as you can, or 5 - 30 seconds.
6.   Repeat twice more.

III. *Dos and Don'ts:*

DO make sure that your legs are together for greater benefit.
DO NOT let the hands support you, for a good work-out of the muscles of the upper back.
DO NOT give up if your legs and chest don't want to lift too far off the floor at first. This will come.

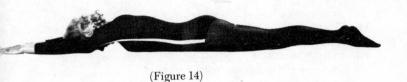

(Figure 14)

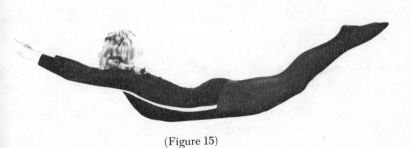

(Figure 15)

The Boat is a gentler version of the more advanced Locust but has most of its benefits without the strain. For the elderly, or people with back problems, the Boat is safe and effective because you are working against gravity and therefore can never go too far.

BOW

I.   *Benefits:*

The Bow ——
- relieves pain from a *slipped disc*.
- tones and firms the muscles of the *abdomen, arms, legs,* and *back*.
- develops and firms the muscles of the *chest* and *bustline*.
- strengthens and limbers up the *spine*.
- reduces weight in *hips* and *buttocks*.
- aids *digestion*.
- improves *posture*.

II.   *Technique:*

1. Lie face down on your abdomen, hands by your side.
2. Bend your knees and bring them close to your buttocks.
3. Grasp your legs at the ankles, one at a time. (Figure 16)
4. Lift your knees off the floor by pulling the ankles *away* from the hands. You will still be tightly holding on, but it is the *away* motion rather than a *down* pull that will do the trick.
5. Lift your head at the same time. (Figure 17)
6. Hold the position for 5-10 seconds at the first, increasing to 30 seconds at 5 seconds a week. Breathe normally.
7. Slowly relax and rest for awhile.
8. Repeat twice more.

III.   *Dos and Don'ts:*

DO come out of the exercise slowly.
DO pull the ankles "up and away" rather than down to get those stubborn knees off the ground.
DON'T collapse in a heap. You will get more exercise for your time.

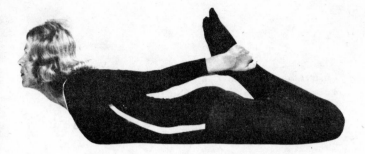

(Figure 16)

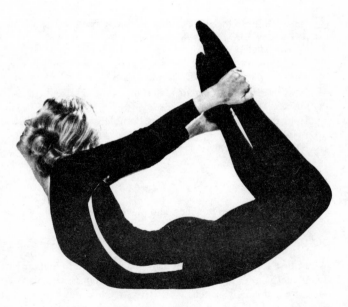

(Figure 17)

This is a demanding but most beneficial exercise and a must in your schedule.

CAMEL

I.   *Benefits:*

The Camel ——
- makes the *spine* flexible and tones it.
- gives a feeling of *energy.*
- improves *posture.*
- benefits rounded *shoulders, hunched backs.*
- beneficial to the *elderly* or people with *spinal injuries,* because it is so gentle.

II. *Technique:*

1. Kneel in an upright position, keeping the legs together, toes pointed back.
2. Place hands on the waist and bend slowly backward, pushing the pelvis forward. (Figure 18)
3. Let the head hang back.
4. Let the right hand hang down over the heel, then the left, and put palms on the feet, if possible. (Figure 19)
5. Pinch the buttocks together, pushing the thighs and pelvis well forward. (Figure 20)
6. Hold this position for as long as possible or from 5 - 30 seconds. Breathe normally.
7. Repeat twice more.

III. *Dos and Don'ts:*

DO remember to keep the chest and pelvis thrust forward for a better bend.
DO NOT press beyond a point of comfort.

At first your hands will only hang slackly down in mid-air and as a beginner you needn't worry about touching your feet. This asana is so gentle and yet gives such an effective stretch to the spine, that anyone over middle age can safely practise it. The Pelvic Stretch is a logical follow-up.

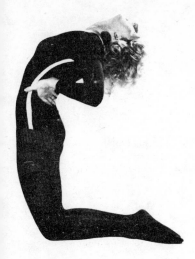

(Figure 18)

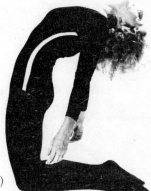

(Figure 19)

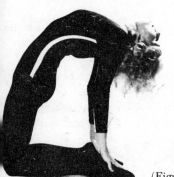

(Figure 20)

CAT STRETCH

I.   *Benefits:*

The Cat Stretch——
- strengthens the *back.*
- reduces *tension.*
- is excellent after *childbirth* to firm sagging female organs.
- tightens the *chin* area.
- stretches the whole *front* of the *body.*
- strengthens the *arms.*

II. *Technique:*

1. Kneel on all fours.
2. Rocking slightly back first, (Figure 21) lower your chest in a sweeping motion, trying to rest the Adam's apple on the floor. (Figure 22)
3. Hold the position for 5 seconds, with most of the weight on the arms.
4. Return to the first position and arch the back in an upward motion rather like an angry, spitting cat. (Figure 23)
5. Hold for 5 seconds, relax.
6. Now bring your right knee towards the head, and touch it if you can. Hold 5 seconds. (Figure 24)
7. Stretch the leg out and up in back, keeping it straight. Hold. Keep the head up and arms straight. (Figure 25)
8. Return the leg slowly to the head. Hold.
9. Relax. Repeat on the other side.
10. Repeat the whole series once more.

III. *Dos and Don'ts:*

DO enjoy the stretching movement of your body. Move slowly and with grace.

DO NOT be discouraged by not getting your knees to your head for awhile. It will come.

The Cat Stretch is a particularly fine exercise for relaxing. It is recommended by gynecologists after childbirth and helps with those vague aches and pains in the lower back and abdominal area.

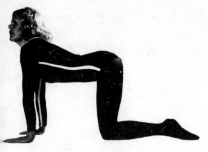

(Figure 21)

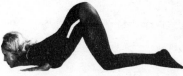

(Figure 22)

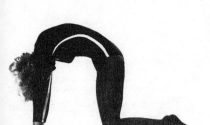

(Figure 23)

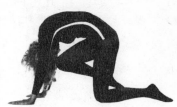

(Figure 24)

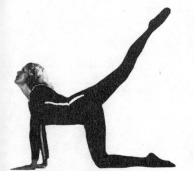

(Figure 25)

CHEST EXPANDER

I.   *Benefits:*

The Chest Expander ——
- builds the *bust* for the ladies and expands the *chest* for the men.
- relieves tension in the *neck, shoulders* and *upper back*.
- acts as a quick *energizer*.
- *relaxes* the whole body.
- firms and reduces a "layered" *tummy*.
- improves *posture*.
- expands the *lungs* and improves *circulation* to the head.

II. *Technique:*

1. Stand straight, feet slightly apart and bring arms forward, palms together. (Figure 26)
2. Bring the arms behind the back in a wide circling motion, knifing the shoulder blades together. Clasp the hands.
3. Letting your head fall back, bend backward as far as you comfortably can, pushing the pelvis forward.
4. Push the clasped hands up toward your head and hold this position for 5 seconds. (Figure 27)
5. Now, staying in the same position, bend slowly forward from the waist, letting the head hang down. Let your body weight pull you down, but do not jerk or bounce. (Figure 28)
6. Hold this position for 10 seconds and keep pushing the hands up towards the head. (Figure 29 — Advanced Pose)
7. Straighten slowly, relax, and then repeat twice more.

III. *Dos and Don'ts:*

DO it often if you are concerned about your bustline.
DON'T close your eyes, in order to keep your balance better.

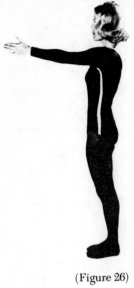

(Figure 26)

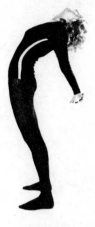

(Figure 27)

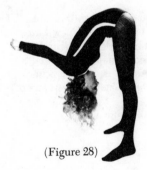

(Figure 28)

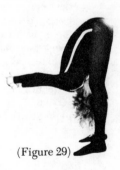

(Figure 29)

The Chest Expander is a wonderful "pick-me-up" after sitting at a desk for hours or when feeling tense and at low ebb.

COBRA

I.   *Benefits:*

The Cobra —
- develops the pectoral muscles of the *bust*.
- stretches and realigns the *vertebrae* of the spinal column. (Beneficial for people with a slipped disc.)
- strengthens the *abdomen* and muscles of the *back*.
- firms and reduces the *buttocks*.
- tones up the *nervous system*.
- aids in *digestion*.
- helps to correct *female disorders*.
- tightens *chin* area.

II.   *Technique:*

1. Lie on your stomach, hands by your side, feet together.
2. Bring the hands, palms down, under the shoulders, a shoulder's width apart. (Figure 30)
3. Lift your head SLOWLY, looking up at the ceiling.
4. When the head is up as far as it will go, and only then, lift the upper shoulders and back, making the muscles of the back do most of the work, rather than the hands.
5. Continue lifting the trunk until you can go no further and still keep the pubic area on the floor. There should be a good arch in the lower spine, but the arms need not be straight. (Figure 31)
6. Hold this position for as long as is comfortable (5-30 seconds).
7. Slowly come out of the Cobra position, feeling the action of each vertebra rolling against the next, and leaving your head up to the very last.
8. Repeat twice more, breathe normally while holding.

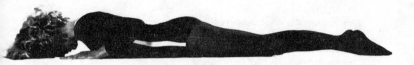

(Figure 30)

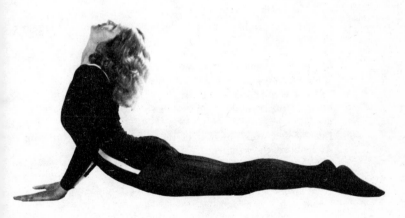

(Figure 31)

III.   *Dos and Don'ts:*

DO make sure that your eyes look upward in their sockets throughout
   going into, holding and coming out of the exercise. Be aware of
   and enjoy the slow movement of your spine, the vertebra-by-
   vertebra massage.

CROSSBEAM

I.   *Benefits:*

The Crossbeam ——
- flattens the *abdominal* region.
- tones and firms the *inner thigh*.
- relieves stiff *backs*.
- stretches the entire *pelvic area*.
- stimulates the *abdominal* organs.
- exercises the *ankles*.

II.   *Technique:*

1. Kneel in an upright position on the floor keeping the feet together.
2. Stretch your right leg out to the right, keeping the knee straight and the toes pointed to the front.
3. Lift both arms out to the side. (Figure 33)
4. Place your right arm onto the right leg, palm up.
5. Bend your body to the right, resting the right ear on the arm. (Figure 34)
6. Lift the left arm slowly over the head, eventually bringing it straight over the right hand, palms touching.
7. Keep your face forward, so that you are peeking through the opening created by the arms. (Figure 35)
8. Hold for a comfortable period (5-30 seconds), breathing normally throughout.

III. *Dos and Don'ts:*

DON'T get discouraged if you are nowhere near the ideal at first. One of the amazing qualities of Yoga is how fast you can improve.

DON'T bend forward from the waist, but make it a sideways stretch.

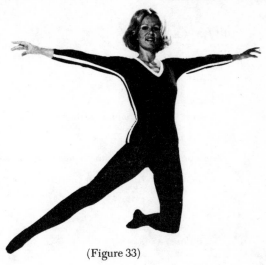

(Figure 33)

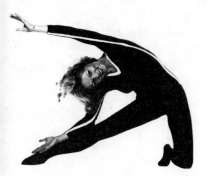

(Figure 34)

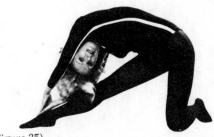

(Figure 35)

CURLING LEAF

I.   *Benefits:*

The Curling Leaf —
- eases *tension,* is wonderfully relaxing.
- acts as an *energy* pick-up.
- improves *circulation* to the *head* which benefits the *complexion.*
- beneficial to *tired legs* and *varicose veins.*

II.   *Technique:*

1. Kneel with legs together.
2. Rest your buttocks on the heels and the top of your hands on the floor, pointing back.
3. Lower your head slowly to the floor, the hands sliding gently back palms up, to lie beside the body.   (Figure 36)
4. Rest your head, turned to the side, on the floor and relax completely with the chest against the knees.
5. Hold for any length of time, the longer the better.

III.   *Dos and Don'ts:*

DO the Curling Leaf any time you need a rest or a pick-up.
DO NOT stick your bottom up in the air but put your whole weight on your legs and heels.

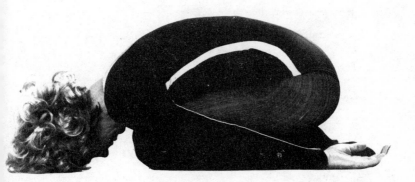

(Figure 36)

This asana is also called "Pose of a Child" and may well be so rest-ful because it is a return-to-the-womb position. It is a most therapeutic pose to assume any time you feel cramped up, tense or tired.

ELBOW EXERCISE

I.   *Benefits:*

The Elbow Exercise ——
- relieves *arthritic* and *bursitic* pain.
- relieves *tension.*
- keeps *arms* flexible.

II. *Technique:*

1. Sit in a comfortably cross-legged position or stand.

2. Bend your elbows and bring them up to shoulder height, the hands curled into a loose fist.   (Figure 37)

3. Now snap the elbows by suddenly thrusting the arms straight. (Figure 38)

4. Relax for a moment and repeat 5 times.

III. *Dos and Don'ts:*

DO make sure that you are really flinging your arms forward as though to throw the hands away.

Yoga is concerned with every part of the body, however negligible it may seem, for these areas are often a seat of tension. This exercise keeps your elbow joints well-greased (and it keeps you from creaking).

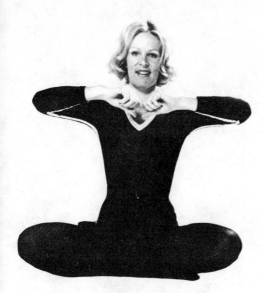

(Figure 37)

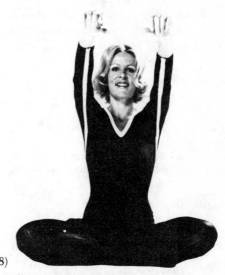

(Figure 38)

EYE EXERCISES

I.   *Benefits:*

The Eye Exercises ——
- relieve *tension, fatigue* and *strain* of the eyes.
- strengthen the *eye* muscles.
- relieve *headaches.*
- give eyes a clear, *shiny* look.
- give a general feeling of *relaxation.*

II.   *Technique:*

1. Sit in a comfortably cross-legged position, look straight ahead.
2. Look as far to the right as is possible without moving the head. Hold 5 seconds.
3. Look to the left. Hold. (Figure 39)
4. Look up under the eyebrows. Hold. (Figure 40)
5. Look down past nose. Hold. (Figure 41)
6. Now imagine a giant clock with the 12 just under the eyebrows and the 6 on the floor immediately in front of you.
7. Look at each digit of this clock for one second, so that your eyes are moving jerkily.
8. Repeat, moving counter-clockwise.
9. Cover your eyes with the palms of both hands for 30 seconds, to rest them. (Figure 42)

Variations:

1. a) Look far away out the windows. Try to look miles toward the horizon. Hold.
    b) Slowly bring your gaze back and look crosseyed at your nose. Hold.
2. Use your imagination:
    e.g., describe semi-circles or diagonals with your eyes.

III. *Dos and Don'ts:*

DO these exercises any time you are very tired or feel that your eyes have been strained, instead of just squeezing the eyes up in the customary fashion.

DO rest the eyes by closing them between each set of exercises.

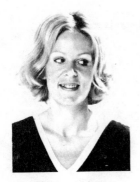

Figure 39)

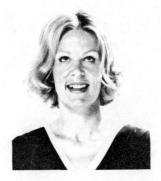

(Figure 40)

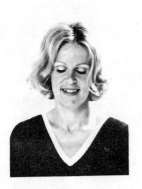

(Figure 41)

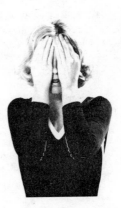

(Figure 42)

The eyes are our most important sense and yet people neglect them greatly by taking them for granted. Eye strain and resulting headaches can be greatly reduced through exercising the eye muscles.

FISH

I. *Benefits:*

The Fish ——

- beneficial for *asthma* and other *respiratory complaints*.
- stimulates the thyroid gland for *weight control*.
- limbers up and relieves *tension* in the *neck* and *upper back*.
- develops the *chest* and *bustline*.
- aids *digestion*.
- relieves painful *piles*.
- improves *circulation* to the *head*.

II. *Technique:*

1. Lie on your back, legs outstretched, arms by your side, palms down. (Figure 43)

2. Pushing down on the elbows, raise your chest off the floor, really arching the back.

3. At the same time pull your head under until you are resting on the very top of it or as close as you can get to the crown. (Figure 44)

4. Shift your weight so that the brunt of it is being borne by the buttocks.

5. Hold the position for 5 - 60 seconds or until you start to be uncomfortable. Breathe normally.

6. Slowly come out of the asana and repeat twice more.

III. *Dos and Don'ts:*

DO put most of your body weight onto the buttocks and elbows.
DO NOT bend your legs at all.

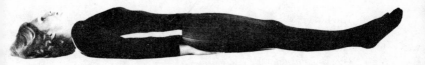

(Figure 43)

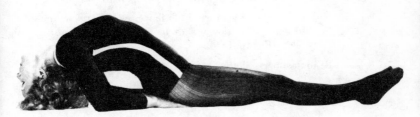

(Figure 44)

The Fish is especially therapeutic for people who suffer from respiratory diseases, since the straightened windpipe greatly facilitates breathing. It also serves as a great "de-tensionizer" of the neck area any time, or after the Shoulderstand and Plough.

FLOWER

I.   *Benefits:*

The Flower —
- eases the pain of *arthritis* and loosens stiff fingers.
- discourages *knobby joints.*
- keeps *hands* looking young.
- improves *circulation.*
- makes and keeps *fingers flexible* for piano-playing, typewriting, needlework, etc.

II.   *Technique:*

1. Sit in a comfortably cross-legged position.

2. Make your hands into tight fists, squeezing hard. (Figure 45)

3. Now visualize that your hand is a flower early in the morning and ever so gently and slowly start to open the hands, *resisting* all the while. (Figure 46)

4. Bend the fingers all the way back. (Figure 47)

5. Reverse the motion and close the hands slowly. The movement must be resisted so that the sinews in the back of the hand stand out.

6. Relax the fingers by moving or shaking them rapidly.

7. Next, with fingers spread apart, press each finger, separately, hard against the palm, holding for 2 seconds each.

8. Repeat the whole series of exercises twice more.

III. *Dos and Don'ts:*

DO the exercises in warm water or oil and you will find a painful effort made much easier with the same benefits.

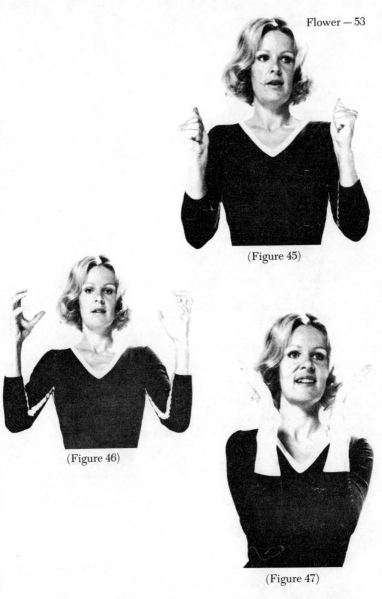

(Figure 45)

(Figure 46)

(Figure 47)

For people who suffer from arthritis it is of great importance that the joints do not stiffen completely. But The Flower also keeps a youthful look for all who are concerned about not letting their age show.

FORWARD BEND (Sitting)

I. *Benefits:*

The sitting Forward Bend —
- strengthens the *abdominal muscles* and tones the *abdominal organs.*
- stretches, limbers up and releases tension in *legs* and *spine.*
- is beneficial to the entire *nervous system.*
- aids *digestion* and *elimination.*
- tones the *kidneys.*
- massages the *heart*
- stretches the *pelvic region* and improves the *circulation* there.
- gives a feeling of *vitality.*

II. *Technique:*

1. Sit on the floor, legs stretched out, feet together and back straight. (Figure 48)
2. Raise your arms parallel to the legs and lean back slightly. (Figure 49)
3. *Slowly* bend forward with a curling motion of the spine, when you have reached your limit without straining or bouncing, grasp tightly that part of your leg which you can comfortably reach. (Figure 50)
4. Now bend your elbows and concentrate on pulling your body forward as well as down, to give a good stretch to the spine.
5. Let your head hang and hold the pose for 5 - 30 seconds, breathing normally.
6. *Eventually* you will be able to bring your head to your knees and grasp the toes instead of the ankles by bringing the elbows to the floor. (Figure 51)
7. Return slowly out of the pose and repeat twice more. .

III. *Dos and Don'ts:*

DO keep your knees straight and remain motionless in this pose, if you do not want to waste your time and effort.
DO NOT bounce to "go further". This will invite injury.

It is more important to give a good forward stretch to the spine, than to push too hard on an at-first reluctant and stiff spine. You will be amazed, however, at your quick downward progress.

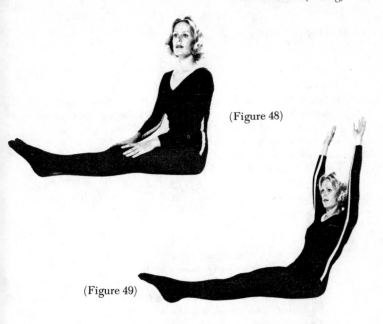

(Figure 48)

(Figure 49)

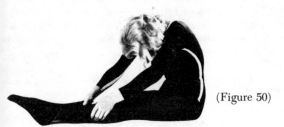

(Figure 50)

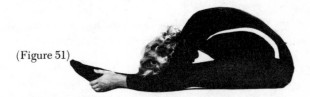

(Figure 51)

FORWARD BEND (Standing)

I.   *Benefits:*

The Forward Bend ——
- releases *tension* in the hamstring muscles and makes the *legs flexible*
- improves *circulation* to the *head*, working on *wrinkles* and *com plexion*, as well as giving a feeling of *alertness*.
- limbers up the *spine*.
- acts as an *energizer*.
- removes *tension* from the *back* and *shoulders*.
- aids *digestion*.
- helps to *reduce excess fat*.

II.   *Technique:*

1. Stand, with the feet slightly apart.
2. Raise your hands slowly above your head. (**Figure 52**)
3. Bend forward slowly from the waist in a curling motion, dropping your head first and then unfurling each vertebra until you can go no further. (**Figure 53**)
4. Keeping your arms beside your ears, let your body hang forward by its own weight for a few seconds. (**Figure 54**)
5. Grasp your ankles, or whatever you can comfortably reach, and dig your chin into the neck.
6. Bend your elbows to the side and give a gentle downward and inward stretch, attempting to get your head as close to the knees as possible. (**Figure 55**)
7. Hold for 5 - 30 seconds.
8. Straighten up very slowly, keeping the arms beside the ears and curling the spine up.
9. Repeat twice more.

III.   *Dos and Don'ts:*

DO NOT bounce or jerk in order to bring your head closer to your knees.

DO NOT worry how close your hands are from the floor, rather how far your head is from your knees.

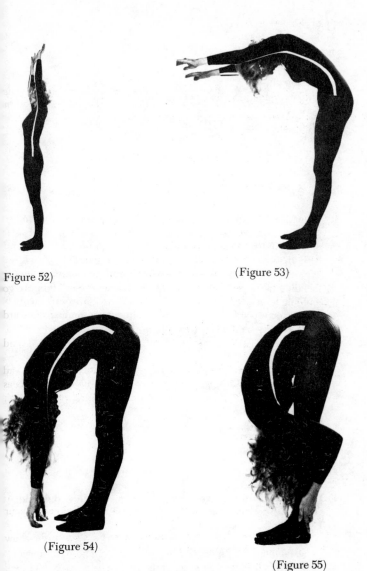

Figure 52)

(Figure 53)

(Figure 54)

(Figure 55)

The Forward Bend Standing works wonders in releasing tension in the back and the hamstring muscles of the legs. The full weight of your hanging body is enough to exercise and loosen these areas and eventually you will be able to touch the floor with your hands.

FOUNTAIN

I. *Benefits:*

The Fountain —
- tightens and reduces weight in the *hips*.
- reduces *waist*.
- improves *circulation* in the *arms*.
- stretches *entire side* of the body.
- relieves *tension*.

II. *Technique:*

1. Stand, feet slightly apart, hands hanging clasped in front of you.
2. Slowly raise the clasped hands over your head and bend as fa back from the waist as you can manage. Hold for a few second (Figure 56)
3. Now describe a circle with your body from the waist up by firs bending to the left, to the front and then to the right, stopping an holding for a few seconds at each location. (Figure 57) (Figure 58
4. Relax and repeat counter-clockwise. Breathe normally throughou Repeat twice more in each direction.

5. *Variations:*
    a) Perform the same steps as above but come up on your toes an balance throughout.
    b) Perform the Fountain without stopping but in very slo motion.
    c) Increase the size of the circles you describe with your body.

III. *Dos and Don'ts:*

DO keep your bottom tucked in when you are bending to the sides t receive the greatest benefits.
DO NOT bend your knees or move your feet.

The Fountain is a specific exercise for those who wish to spot re move weight. It gives you a delightful sensation of stretching and therefore tension-reducing as well.

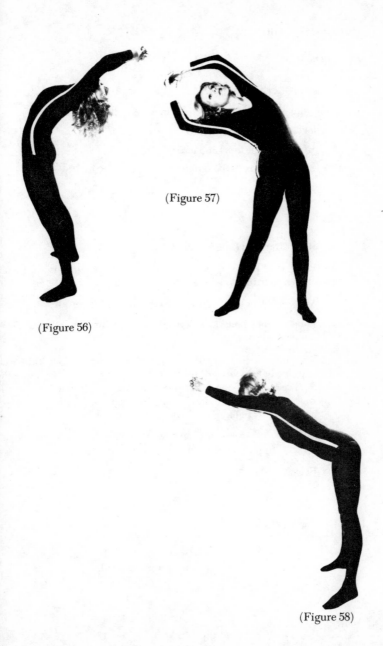

(Figure 57)

(Figure 56)

(Figure 58)

HANDS-TO-WALL

I. *Benefits:*

The Hands-To-Wall Pose ——

- tightens and firms the pectoral muscles of the *bustline*.
- develops the *bust*.
- strengthens the *arms* and *wrists*.
- releases *tension* in the *shoulders*.

II. *Technique:*

1. Stand straight, facing a wall.

2. Place your palms against the wall, fingers pointing toward each other and barely touching.

3. Move an arm's length away from the wall. (Figure 59)

4. Keeping your body in a perfectly straight line throughout, slowly bend the elbows.

5. Press only the palms, rather than the whole hand, against the wall and slowly lean forward resisting the whole time. Slowly bring the forehead against the wall. Be sure that you do not bend at the waist, pushing the buttocks out, but that your body remains an unbroken, straight line. (Figure 60)

6. Hold for 5 - 15 seconds and return just as slowly, resisting the movement, pushing with the palms.

7. Relax.

III. *Dos and Don'ts:*

DO make sure that your body is straight from the shoulders down, by placing yourself an arm's length from the wall.

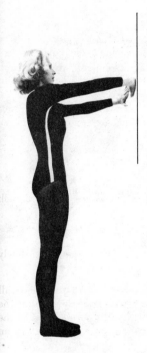

(Figure 59)

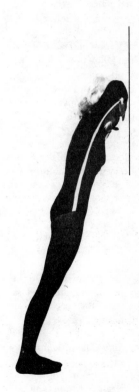

(Figure 60)

HEADSTAND - WALK-UP

I.   *Benefits:* Owing to the reversal of the normal upright position, the following benefits are derived from the Headstand:

- *circulation* is greatly improved to areas which normally get little i) *brain,* ii) *heart,* iii) *pelvis,* iv) *spinal cord.*
- the *nervous system* is toned owing to balancing and circulation.
- *abdominal organs,* which normally sag or prolapse, are pulled into original position.
- *stomach muscles* are firmed and strengthened.
- *sinus fluids* are now permitted to flow downward.
- the *endocrine, pituitary*-and *pineal glands* are stimulated into normal action.
- *energy* and a general feeling of *alertness* are experienced.
- strenghthens the *lungs.*
- *digestion* and *elimination* are improved.
- the following ailments are removed or their condition is improved:
   a) insomnia
   b) colds and sore throats
   c) palpitations
   d) bad breath
   e) headaches
   f) asthma
   g) varicose veins
   h) lack of sexual interest

II.   *Technique:*

1. Make sure that you have adequate support for your head: a carpet with underfelt or a blanket folded in four.
2. Kneel on the carpet or in front of the blanket with your toes tucked under.
3. Clasp your hands tightly and place them on the floor with the elbows not more, nor less, than a shoulder's width apart. (Figure 61)
4. Place the very top of the head on the floor, disregarding the hands for now.
5. Now pull the folded hands against the back of the head *on the floor.* The little fingers will be under the curvature of the head. (Figure 62)
6. Push your bottom straight up and with the knees absolutely straight throughout, slowly tippy-toe up towards your head. The object is to make the back straight. (Figure 63, Figure 64)

7. When you can go no further, hold the position for as long as comfort permits, then slowly walk down again.
8. Relax with your head down for awhile.
9. Repeat twice more, or as often as you wish to get the feel of balance. (Figures 64, 65, 66 — Advanced Poses)

III. *Dos and Don'ts:*

DO clasp your hands very tightly and take your rings off to prevent slipping and undue strain on the arms.

DO NOT let your elbows flare out or press against the head. For a perfect tripod they are a shoulder's width apart.

DO put the crown of the head on the floor. Contrary to what you have learned in calisthenics classes, it is not the hairline nor the back of the head that will support you longest and most comfortably. Eventually you may be able to stand on your head from 5 - 30 minutes.

DO NOT put the back of the head against the hands but rather bring the hands against the head. Do a little bit of nestling there to make sure you will be comfortable.

DO keep the knees very straight to make possible a straight back.

DO NOT, repeat, DO *NOT* push up on your toes to get you up into the Headstand. Unless the toes lift off *by themselves* you are not ready to bring the legs up. Even when you are ready, practice balance by hugging the knees to the chest for awhile. The hardest part of the Headstand Proper is bringing the legs up and that is mainly done by strong abdominal muscles. The Headstand is a feat of strength rather than skill.

DO practice the Cobra and the Bow to make the neck strong and flexible. This is especially true for round-shouldered people.

DO practice the Pump, Sit-Up and Abdominal Lift to strengthen tummy muscles if you topple over as soon as you try to straighten your legs.

DO take your time and be patient with yourself. The Headstand is one of the most difficult poses in Yoga and will take time, strength, flexibility and balance to accomplish. Develop these skills first. The "Walk-Up" will prepare you in all respects for eventually doing the Headstand and it is an excellent exercise in its own right.

(Figure 61)

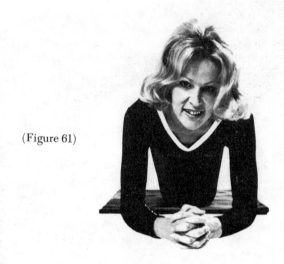

(Figure 62)

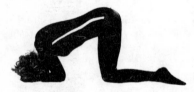

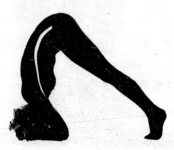

(Figure 63)

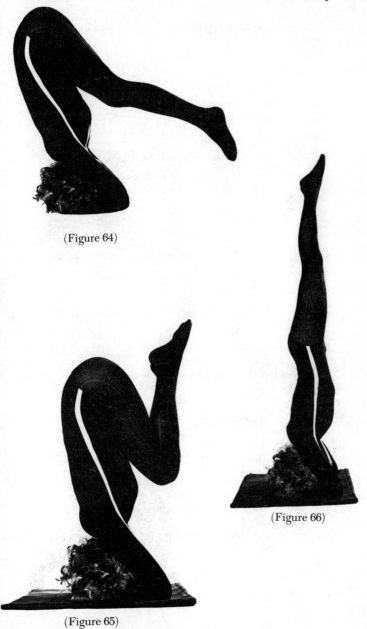

(Figure 64)

(Figure 65)

(Figure 66)

JAPANESE SITTING POSITION

I. *Benefits:*

The Japanese Sitting Position ——
- removes tension from the *ankles.*

- stretches the *upper thighs.*

- limbers up the *knee joint.*

- is beneficial for *varicose veins* and *tired legs.*

- removes *tension* from the whole foot, particularly the *arch.*

II. *Technique:*

1. Kneel in an upright position, feet together, toes pointing back.

2. Slowly lower your buttocks onto the heels, using your hands for support, if you wish.

3. Relax, placing your weight onto the heels, keeping the back straight. (Figure 67)

4. Place your hands on your thighs.

5. As you improve, point the toes together, let the heels fall apart and nestle in this "seat".

III. *Dos and Don'ts:*

DO sit in the "Japanese Sitting Position" whenever possible.
DO keep your back straight.

The floor acts as an exercising machine whenever you are on it.

DO use it rather than your "comfortable" furniture which aids and abets you in slouching.

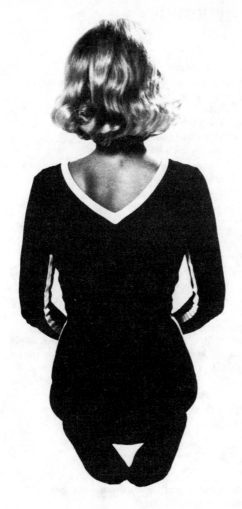

(Figure 67)

After an initial stiffness goes away, and that will happen quickly, this Yoga Posture has a very beneficial effect on your muscles and nerves.

KNEE AND THIGH STRETCH

I. *Benefits:*

The Knee and Thigh Stretch ——
- is very beneficial for *bladder and urinary problems.*
- keeps the *prostate gland* healthy.
- tones *kidneys.*
- firms and reduces weight in *inner thighs.*
- gives new vitality to *tired legs.*
- helps to prepare women for *childbirth.*
- stimulates function of the *ovaries* and helps to regulate *menstrual periods.*
- relieves *sciatic pain.*

II. *Technique:*

1. Sit on the floor, legs outstretched, back straight.
2. Bend your knees to the side and bring the soles of your feet together. (Figure 68)
3. Clasp your fingers tightly around the toes and gently pull the feet as close to the body as you can, possibly touching the perineum. (Figure 69)
4. Now with a great effort of will, widen the thighs and attempt to bring the knees to the floor by pulling up on the toes.
5. Hold the position for as long as you can -- from 5 - 30 seconds. The secret here lies in breathing normally as you are holding. (Figure 70)
6. Relax by stretching the legs out and shaking them if you wish.
7. Repeat twice more; or 4 times more if you are really concerned about your health problem or flabby inner thighs.

III. *Dos and Don'ts:*

DO clasp your fingers tightly around the toes to give you a good hold and to prevent slipping.

DO NOT push the knees forcibly with your hands. You can accomplish much more by your will.

DO NOT be discouraged if your knees look like craggy mountains for awhile. With patient perseverance you have an excellent chance of eventually laying the knees on the floor.

DO try to relax, even as you are holding.

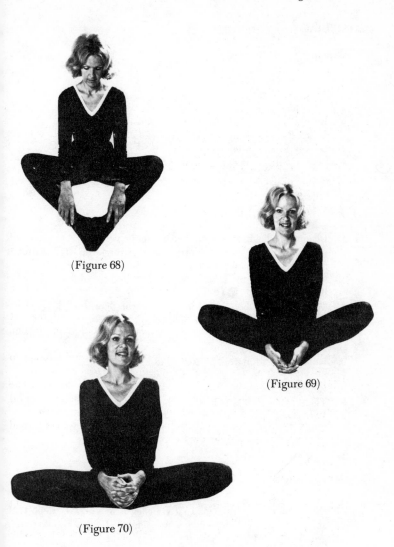

(Figure 68)

(Figure 69)

(Figure 70)

The Knee and Thigh Stretch is a demanding but very important exercise. It is a pose customarily adopted by the Indian cobbler, who has been found by Medical Authorities to be practically free of urinary and bladder complaints.

LEG-OVER

I. *Benefits:*

The Leg-Over ——
- reduces *fat*.
- massages and stimulates *liver, spleen, pancreas*.
- aids *digestion* and relieves *gastritis*.
- tones and firms *abdominal organs*.
- relieves sprains in *lower back* and *hip*.

II. *Technique:*

1. Lie on your back, arms stretched out to the side.
2. Lift your right leg slowly until it points straight up. Do not bend the knee throughout. (Figure 71)
3. Move the leg to the left across the body and try to lower it to the floor.
4. Make sure that *both* shoulders stay on the floor, even if you have to grip a chair leg with your right hand.
5. When the leg has gone as far as it will go, turn your head to the right. (Figure 72)
6. Hold the position from 5 - 20 seconds.
7. Slowly bring the leg up and then lower it.
8. Repeat with the other leg.
9. Then repeat with both legs together. (Figure 73)
10. *Variation:*
    a) Bend both legs at the knee and bring them to the side.

III. *Dos and Don'ts:*

DO NOT roll over to the side that your leg is moving to. Keep both shoulders on the floor to give your spine a delightful spiral stretch.
DO turn your head in the opposite direction of the leg.

The Leg-Over is gentle enough to be safely practiced even by the elderly. It gives a maximum stretch to the spine with a minimum of effort.

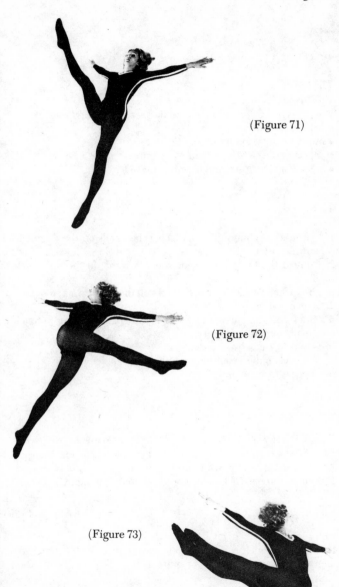

(Figure 71)

(Figure 72)

(Figure 73)

LION

I. *Benefits:*

The Lion ——
- reduces *tension* in the *face* area.
- tightens and firms the muscles of the *face, neck* and *throat.*
- reduces a *double chin.*
- smoothes *lines* and *wrinkles.*
- improves the *circulation* and *complexion.*
- relieves a *sore throat* and improves the *voice.*

II. *Technique:*

1. Sit in a kneeling position, placing the hands on the thighs, palms down. (**Figure 74**)
2. Spread the fingers and slide them forward till the tips touch the floor.
3. Bend your body forward, buttocks off the heels, arms straight.
4. Open your eyes as wide as possible.
5. Stick your tongue out as far as it will go, attempting to touch the tip of your chin. (**Figure 75**)
6. Hold 15 seconds.
7. Sit back, pull in your tongue and relax completely.
8. Repeat twice more.

III. *Dos and Don'ts:*

DO stick your tongue out completely for a good stretch.
DO NOT be surprised if you have a gagging sensation for awhile.
DO the Lion at the sun with the eyes closed.
DO enjoy the marvellous feeling of tension draining away when you sit back.

The Lion is a must in anyone's life: for beauty for the ladies, tension for the men. It gives your complexion a new glow and erases those tired lines. It can be done anywhere, or even, perhaps, if you are angry at someone. That may be quite therapeutic.

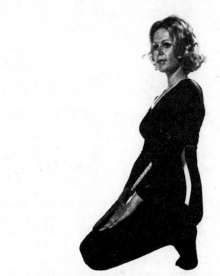

(Figure 74)

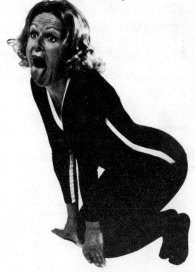

(Figure 75)

MOUNTAIN

I.   *Benefits:*

The Mountain ——
- tones the *nervous system*.
- aids *digestion* and removes *constipation*.
- tones and firms *abdominal muscles* and *trunk*.
- strengthens the *spine*.
- if coupled with proper breathing, strengthens the *lungs* and oxygenates the *bloodstream*.
- reduces *tension*.

II.   *Technique:*

1. Sit in a comfortably cross-legged position, the back straight.
2. Bring the palms of both hands together in front of your chest, as if praying. (**Figure 76**)
3. Pressing the palms firmly together, slowly stretch the arms above the head.
4. Stretch the finger-tips toward the ceiling in a tremendous stretch. (**Figure 77**)
5. Hold the posture for 5 - 30 seconds, breathing normally.
6. Slowly bring the hands down.
7. Relax.
8. This can also be done as a deep breathing exercise.

III. *Dos and Don'ts:*

DO keep your back straight to give it a very therapeutic stretch.
DO NOT hold your breath.

The Mountain is a most deceptive pose. Those who scoffed at a demonstration had to admit it was a demanding exercise. Done properly, the stretch, however, is exhilarating.

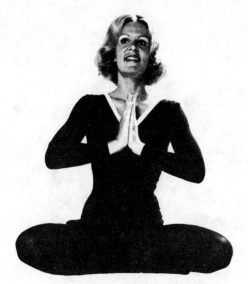

(Figure 76)

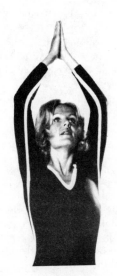

(Figure 77)

NECK ROLLS

I. *Benefits:*

The Neck Rolls ——
- reduce deep-seated tension in *neck area*.
- relieve *stiff neck* and often *headaches*.
- help to relax the entire body -- excellent for *insomnia*.
- reduce *double chin*.

II. *Technique:*

1. Sit, shoulders back, in a comfortably cross-legged position, or on a chair.

2. Let your head drop slowly until it hangs limply as a rag-doll's. Hold.

3. Bring the head up and, keeping shoulders straight, let your head fall back. How far you can bring it back depends on how tense you are. (Figure 78)

4. Keep mouth closed, teeth together. Hold.

5. Hang your head to the side, looking up. Hold. Repeat on other side. (Figure 80)

6. Pretending to be a rag-doll, let your head droop and roll it gently, but firmly, first to the right, then the back, to the left and forward again. There should be no conscious control, just a limp lolling of the head in a *full* circle.

7. Repeat on the other side. Repeat the full circle several times.

III. *Comment:*

As a quick relaxer and pick-me-up, the Neck Rolls are unique. With your eyes closed you will experience a marvellously relaxing sensation. Be sure to do the exercise slowly and with care, rolling gently over the inevitable sore spots. A gritty, gravelly sound may be heard at first, but will gradually disappear with practice, as the neck joints are being lubricated. One of the first signs of age is a sort of "fusing" of the neck to the spine.

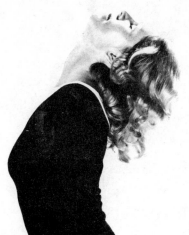

(Figure 78)

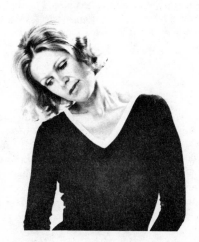

(Figure 80)

PELVIC STRETCH

I.   *Benefits:*

The Pelvic Stretch ——
- removes *tension*.
- stretches and firms *thighs, hips* and *abdomen*.
- strengthens *back* and *legs*.
- has a stimulating effect on *glands* and *abdominal organs*.
- limbers up the *spine*.
- develops the pectoral muscles of the *bustline* and expands *chest*
- improves *postures*.
- firms and removes fatty deposits on the back of the *legs*.
- stretches and removes tension from *feet* and *ankles*.

II.   *Technique:*

1. Kneel, resting on the heels, legs together. (Figure 81)
2. Place your right hand on the floor behind you, elbow straight, fingers pointing back.
3. Place the left hand on the other side, having both hands straight down from the shoulders.
4. Let your head hang back. (Figure 82)
5. Push up on the pelvis as far as it will go and hold for 5 - 30 seconds. (Figure 83)
6. Slowly lower yourself and come forward into the Curling Leaf: head resting on the floor, chest against the knees, buttocks resting on the heels, arms resting by your side. (Figure 36)
7. Repeat, angling your hands further back each time, but always return to the Curling Leaf. (Figure 84)
8. Perform three times.

III. *Dos and Don'ts:*
DO NOT forget to push your pelvis up, so that the buttocks are no longer resting on the heels. The whole front of your body should be describing an arch.
DO bring the body forward after each pose to off-set the extreme backward stretch.

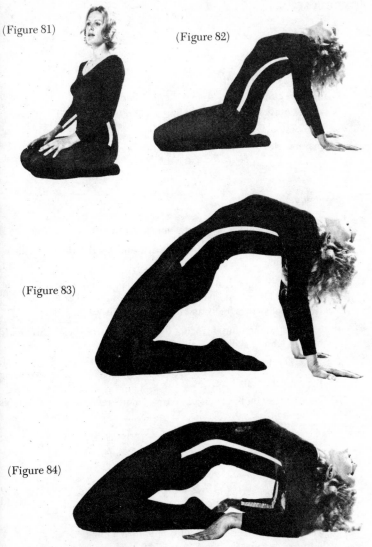

(Figure 81)

(Figure 82)

(Figure 83)

(Figure 84)

Eventually you will be able to lower yourself onto your elbows and shoulders. This asana is especially beneficial for women. Together with the Forward Bend it can alleviate a lot of the vague aches and pains common to females.

PENDULUM

I. *Benefits:*

The Pendulum ——
- relieves pain of *bursitis.*
- improves circulation to *head* and *upper body.*
- relieves *tension* and gives a feeling of *energy.*
- improves *posture.*
- tones muscles of *shoulders* and *upper back.*

II. *Technique:*

1. Stand, feet comfortably apart, your left hand at the waist. (Figure 85)

2. Bend slowly forward from the waist and let the right arm hang limply down.

3. Swing your right arm like a pendulum in a long oval in front of your feet. It is important here that the arm is not stiffly directed by you but swings freely and limply. (Figure 86)

4. Slowly straighten up, bringing the right arm over-head. Stretch it back as far as it will go. Hold. Relax. (Figure 87)

5. Repeat with the other arm.

6. Repeat with both arms.

7. Perform the whole exercise 2 - 3 times more, reversing the direction of the oval.

III. *Dos and Don'ts:*

DO keep the knees straight.
DO NOT move the arm stiffly.

The Pendulum is deceptively simple for people without problems in that area, but for the tense person, or the sufferer of bursitis, this asana gives maximum relief with a minimum of discomfort.

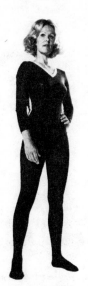

(Figure 85)

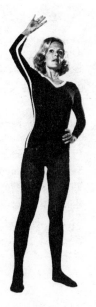

(Figure 87)

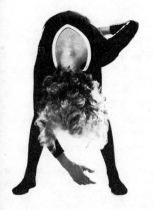

(Figure 86)

PERFECT POSTURE

I.   *Benefits:*

The Perfect Posture —
- is ideal for prolonged *sitting* (meditation).
- is relaxing for the *entire body*.
- stretches and tones *legs* and *lower back*.
- is beneficial to *bladder* and *urinary tracts*.

II.   *Technique:*

1.   Sit with both legs extended and spread apart.

2.   Bring the sole of the right foot against the thigh of the left leg, resting the right knee on the floor.   (Figure 88)

3.   Bend the left leg and, grabbing the toes with both hands, gently lift the left foot onto the right foot.

4.   Adjust for comfort by having the ankles beside, rather than on top of, each other. Snuggle the toes of the left foot into the cleft created by the thigh and calf of the right leg.   (Figure 89)

5.   Keep your spine straight and try to keep both knees as close to the floor as possible.

6.   Rest in this position until the beginning of discomfort.

7.   Change feet and try again.

III.   *Comments:*

As with most yoga exercises, the Perfect Posture cannot be forced. Some can assume it at once (these are usually double-jointed) and for others it may take a year or so. Since the muscles of the knee are easily strained, it does not pay to be overly ambitious. However, do keep at it, even if your knees are sticking out at odd angles, because eventually this is a most comfortable and healthy sitting position. While just sitting, you are exercising madly.

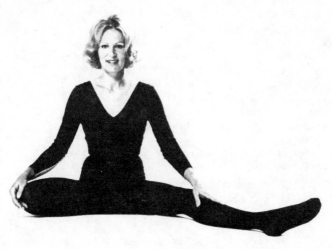

(Figure 88)

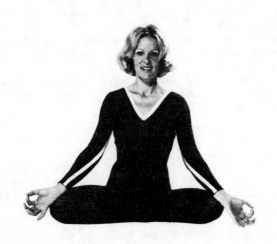

(Figure 89)

PLOUGH

I. *Benefits:*

The Plough ——
- makes the *spine* supple.
- stimulates the *thyroid gland* for weight control.
- strengthens and firms the *abdomen.*
- slims and firms *thighs* and *hips.*
- relieves deep-seated *tension* and *headaches.*
- tones up the *nervous system.*
- improves *circulation.*
- massages such abdominal organs as the *liver, spleen, pancreas* and *kidneys.*
- acts as an *energy* pick-me-up.
- strengthens the *neck.*
- helps to reduce the *bust.*

II. *Techniques:*

1. Lie on your back on the floor, legs outstretched, arms extended by your side, palms down.
2. Slowly lift your legs by tightening the abdominal and leg muscles.
3. Push down on your hands, making them hollow or tent-like and raise your buttocks and lower back. (**Figure 90**)
4. Bring your legs over your head, attempting to touch the floor behind you with the toes, by bending at the waist. Keep your knees straight. (**Figure 91**)
5. Hold the position, even if your feet are nowhere near the floor, for as long as you comfortably can or up to a minute.
6. Breathe normally.
7. Slowly come out of the pose by bending your knees, but straighten the legs when they are perpendicular to the floor. (**Figure 92**, **Figure 93** — Advanced Pose)

III. *Dos and Don'ts:*

DO NOT become discouraged if you can only raise your bottom a couple of inches off the floor. Simply go as far as you can, hold it there and repeat this action several times. The holding process strengthens and prepares the proper muscles for the exercise.
DO keep your knees straight throughout.
DO NOT lift your head as you lower your legs.
DO breathe normally. It will get easier with practice.

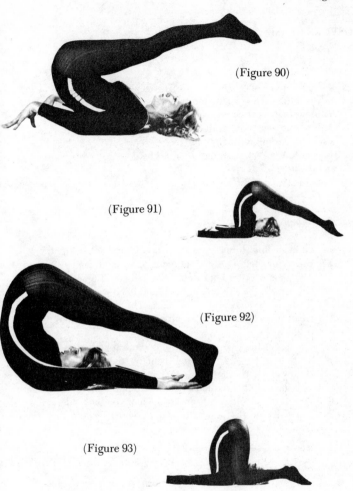

(Figure 90)

(Figure 91)

(Figure 92)

(Figure 93)

DO place your legs on a low bench behind you, if you experience a breathless sensation at first. This will pass with familiarity of the pose.

You will be astounded at your fast progression in the Plough. Even elderly people can comfortably bring the toes to the floor in a relatively short time. This asana gives a delightful, relaxing stretch to the spine that has been unnaturally compressed through years of improper use. It is one of my most favourite exercises.

POSTURE CLASP

I. *Benefits:*

The Posture Clasp —
- eases the pain of *bursitis*.
- improves *posture* and *rounded shoulders*.
- firms and strengthens the *upper arms*.
- eases tension in the *shoulders*.
- exercises muscles around *shoulder blades* and *upper back*.
- oils *shoulder joints*.
- expands the *chest*.

II. *Technique:*

1. Sit in a comfortably cross-legged position, back straight.
2. Bring your left hand behind your back, palm facing out and try to wriggle it up your back as far as it will go. (Figure 94)
3. Lift your right hand straight up and bend it at the elbow, bringing the hand to the centre of the back. This pose is also called the Cow Head pose because of the elbow sticking up to look like a horn. (Figure 95)
4. Try to get the two hands close enough together to interlock with the fingers, by gently inching them together.
5. Hold the position for 10 - 30 seconds and try a gentle upward pull with the right hand, then a downward pull with the left. (Figure 96)
6. Repeat on the other side and twice more on both sides.
7. You will find that one side is much more flexible than the other. Concentrate on the stiffer one.

III. *Dos and Don'ts:*

DO keep your back straight and you will have better success.
DO NOT strain beyond a point of comfort.
DO use a kerchief if your fingers are too far apart. (Figure 96a)

The Posture Clasp is a quick tension-reducer, especially if you spend a lot of your time hunched over a desk. It improves your posture, which in turn improves your health, particularly a tense and brittle back.

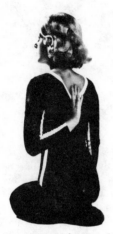

(Figure 94)

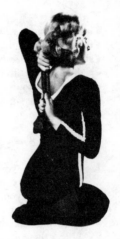

(Figure 96a)

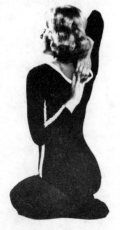

(Figure 95)

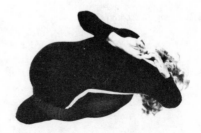

(Figure 96)

PUMP

I. *Benefits:*

The Pump ——
- improves *circulation* throughout the body.
- firms and strengthens *abdomen.*
- strengthens *back muscles.*
- tightens and firms *derriere.*
- reduces fat around the *middle.*
- tones and massages *abdominal organs.*
- relieves *flatulence* (stomach gas) and aids *digestion.*

II. *Technique:*

1. Lie prone on your back, arms very close by your side, palms down.
2. With legs outstretched and together, push down on your palms.
3. *Slowly* raise your legs, keeping the knees straight. (Figure 97) Take a total of 15 seconds to bring them perpendicular to the floor.
4. Hold and rest with the legs up. (Figure 98)
5. Lower them just as slowly, moving slower as you come closer to the floor. (Figure 99)
6. Repeat twice more, or more often if you are really concerned about flattening the tummy.
7. *Variation:*
    a) Lie on back, etc., as above. Slowly raise your legs to a 30° angle off the floor. Hold ten seconds. Now raise the legs to a 60° angle and hold 10 seconds. Bring the legs perpendicular to the floor and lower slowly.
    b) Directly after child birth or if you have very weak abdominal muscles, start by raising the legs one at a time.

III. *Dos and Don'ts:*

DO move very slowly in order to receive the greatest benefits. The closer you are to the floor, the slower you must move.

DO NOT bend your knees or lift your head as you come out of the Pump.

DO NOT hold your breath.

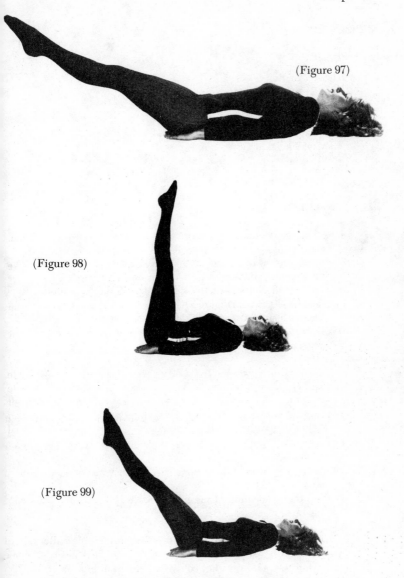

(Figure 97)

(Figure 98)

(Figure 99)

As a specific for tightening the tummy muscles, the Pump is a MUST. It is a demanding exercise but it also produces satisfying results.

ROCKN' ROLLS

I.   *Benefits:*

The Rockn' Rolls —
- act as an excellent *warm-up* and *energizer.*
- limber up the *spine.*
- strengthen the *abdominal muscles.*
- massage and reduce *tension* in the *neck* and *spine.*
- are beneficial to the *liver* and *spleen.*
- aid *digestion* and *elimination.*

II.   *Technique:*

1.   Sit on the floor, knees bent.
2.   Clasp your hands under the knees.
3.   Bring your head as close to the knees as possible and keep it there throughout. (Figure 100)
4.   Rock gently back onto the spine, keeping the back rounded and the legs together. (Figure 101)
5.   Establish an easy rhythm in rocking back and forth. (Figure 102)
6.   Repeat 12 times or up to a minute.
7.   Remember to breathe.

III. *Dos and Don'ts:*

DO start the whole exercise on your back if you are a bit timid about rocking back from a sitting position.

DO the Rockn' Rolls any time you want to get the kinks out of your body.

DO keep your head close to your knees, to have a rounded spine to rock on.

DO use the momentum of the first backward rock to return forward again.

The Rockn' Rolls are my husband's favourite exercise after a hard day at the office. He very wisely does them right after he comes home and before supper, instead of collapsing in a heap in front of the T.V. He is confident that they unwind him and help him to face the rest of the evening.

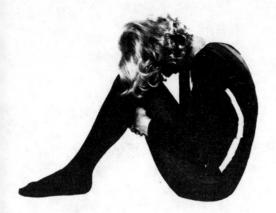

(Figure 100)

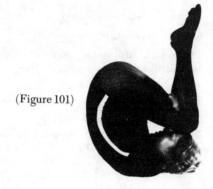

(Figure 101)

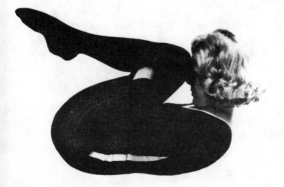

(Figure 102)

SCALP EXERCISE

I.   *Benefits:*

The Scalp Exercise ——
- improves *circulation* to *scalp.*

- removes *tension.*

- makes hair healthy and shiny and, therefore, helps to *prevent loss of hair.*

II.   *Technique:*

1.   Sit in a comfortably cross-legged position.

2.   Get hold of your hair in big fistfulls.

3.   Keeping the fists pressed against the scalp, yank the hair forward, backward and to the sides in fairly rapid motion. (Figure 103)

4.   Now release the hair and place all ten fingers of your spread-apart hands on the scalp, as though to shampoo.

5.   Keep the fingers pressed firmly against the scalp and move it in all directions as above, rather than moving each individual finger.

6.   Repeat several times. (Figure 103a)

III. *Dos and Don'ts:*

DO be sure that you have lots of hair in your fists, otherwise it will hurt.
DO hold the hair close to the scalp.

The Scalp Exercise gives a lovely, tingly feeling to your scalp and removes the tight band of tension.

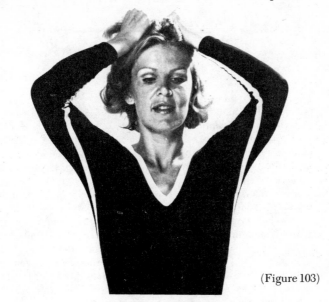

(Figure 103)

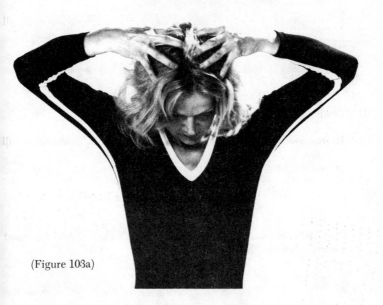

(Figure 103a)

SHOULDERSTAND

I.   *Benefits:*

The Shoulderstand ——

- is a cure-all for most *common ailments.*
- improves the *circulation* to such important areas as the *brain*, the *spine*, the *pelvic area;* these are areas which, due to an upright position, rarely receive a good supply of rich, newly-oxygenated blood.
- presses the chin against the thryroid gland which stimulates it and *reduces excess fat.*
- tones up the central *nervous system* and soothes it (tension, insomnia, inability) and is a marvellous rejuvenator.
- has a beneficial effect on the *hormone-producing glands of the body.*
- relieves *palpitation, breathlessness, bronchitis, throat ailments and asthma* due to increased circulation to neck and chest.
- relieves pressure on abdominal organs due to body-inversion, which, in turn, regulates the *digestive processes,* frees the body of *toxins* and increases the *energy-level.*
- is beneficial for *urinary disorders, menstrual troubles* and *piles.*
- relieves *varicose veins* and *aching legs.*
- gives new vitality to people who suffer from *anemia* or *lack of energy*
- relaxes *whole body.*
- rejuvenates the *sexual glands* and *organs.*
- stretches the *spine.*
- strengthens and firms the muscles of the *back, legs, neck* and *abdomen*

II.   *Technique:*

1.   Lie on the floor, legs out-stretched, hands close by your side, palms down.
2.   Slowly lift your legs by tensing the abdominal and leg muscles, until they are perpendicular to the floor.
3.   Press down on your hands, making them hollow or tent-like. (Figure 104)
4.   Raise your buttocks and lower back and grasp yourself around the waist, with the thumbs around the front of the body. DO NOT let the elbows flare out. (Figure 105)
5.   Straighten the legs and tuck the bottom in as much as balance permits.
6.   If you are balancing well, then grasp yourself up higher on the rib-cage and tuck your bottom in. (Figure 106)

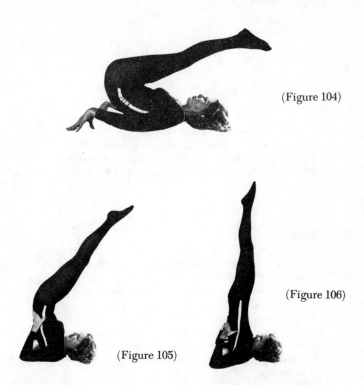

(Figure 104)

(Figure 106)

(Figure 105)

7. Stretch your legs and point your toes. Hold the position from 10 - 60 seconds, as a beginner. Gradually work up to 3 minutes. Breathe normally throughout.

III. *Dos and Don'ts:*

DO be patient with yourself. The important thing is to be up there at all, even if it is not ramrod straight at the start.

DO NOT get alarmed if you feel slightly dizzy or heady at first. It is quite normal and can be blamed on the sudden dilation of the blood vessels.

The Sanskrit translation of the word "sarvang" is "all parts" and means that the Headstand (or Sarvangasana) is the most marvellous of exercises because the whole body receives benefits in this position. I, personally, practice the Shoulderstand every day and miss it's benefits the next day if I don't. How very nice to have one exercise that combines so many benefits in it's action.

SITTING WARRIOR

I.   *Benefits:*

The Sitting Warrior —
- is beneficial for *flat feet.*
- is recommended for 10 minutes when the *legs* are *tired.*
- relieves *rheumatic pain* in the *knees.*
- forms proper *arches* and eases tension in them.
- relieves pain in the *heels* and pain from *calcaneal spurs.*
- relieves the *feeling* of a *heavy stomach* and is safe to do immediately after eating.

II.   *Technique:*

1.   Kneel in an upright position, knees together, the feet a foot and a half apart. (Figure 107)
2.   Slowly lower your body to sit between the feet *on the floor.* Use your hands for support if you wish. (Figure 107a)
3.   Straighten your back and keep the toes pointed straight back.
4.   Place your wrists on the knees, palms down. (Figure 108)
5.   Hold for 30 seconds, breathing deeply.
6.   Now clasp your fingers and stretch your arms straight up, palms facing up.
7.   Hold for 30 seconds.
8.   Relax.

III. *Dos and Don'ts:*

DO relax in the pose. It is marvellously resting after awhile.
DO NOT give up if sitting with the feet apart is difficult at first. Cross your ankles for awhile and sit on the feet this way. Gradually move your feet further and further apart.

Many people who have to be on their feet a lot have found this pose very beneficial. In its advanced form, you lie back onto your shoulders from the sitting position. That pose is called the Reclining Warrior.

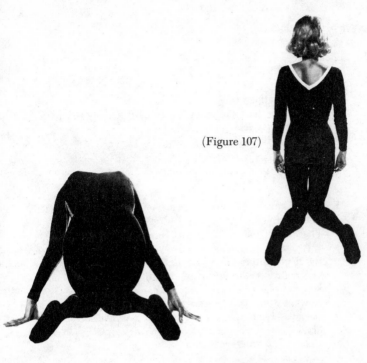

(Figure 107)

(Figure 107a)

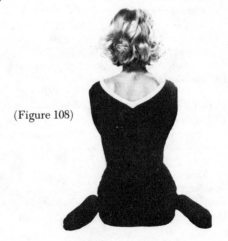

(Figure 108)

SIT-UP

I.   *Benefits:*

The Sit-Up —
• gently strengthens *back*.
• is one of the best exercising for firming, toning and flattening the *abdominal muscles*.
• firms and tightens *derriere*.

II.   *Technique:*

1.   Lie on your back, knees bent *just* enough to permit the whole foot to touch the floor.
2.   Place your hands on the thighs. (Figure 109)
3.   Lift your head slowly and raise your upper body to a 30° angle off the floor, sliding the hands up the legs. Depending on the length of your arms, the fingertips should barely be touching the bent knee-cap.
4.   Keeping your back as straight as possible, hold the position 5 - 30 seconds. (Figure 110)
5.   Slowly lower your trunk. Relax.
6.   Repeat 3 - 5 times more.

III.   *Dos and Don'ts:*

DO NOT go much further than a 30° angle. If the exercise comes too easily, if the rectal muscles of the abdomen are not standing out in a taut ridge, you may be sure that you are doing it wrong.
DO breathe normally.

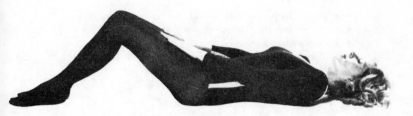

(Figure 109)

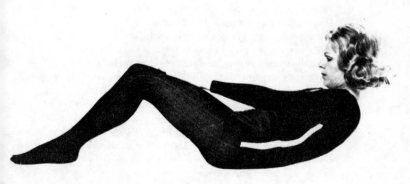

(Figure 110)

The Sit-Up is an excellent tummy and paunch conditioner and flattener. Unfortunately, the tummy muscle exercises are all demanding poses but give quick results if practiced regularly.

SPONGE

I.   *Benefits:*

The Sponge ——
- promotes deep *muscular relaxation.*
- deeply *relaxes* the *nervous system.*
- restores *peace of mind.*
- results in a reduction of *anxiety* or "nerves" through the release of tension.
- is a marvellous, *energy-recharger.*

II.   *Technique:*

1. Lie on the floor, legs slightly apart, arms limply by your side. (Figure 111)
2. Point your toes away from you and hold for 5 seconds. Relax.
3. Pull the toes up towards the body, bending at the ankle. Hold. Relax.
4. Pull your heels up two inches on the floor and then straighten the legs, pushing the back of the knees firmly against the floor. Hold. Relax.
5. Point the toes toward each other and pull the heels under and up, keeping the legs straight. Hold. Relax.
6. Pinch your buttocks together. Hold. Relax.
7. Pull your abdomen in and up as far as possible. Hold. Relax.
8. Arch the spine back, pushing the chest out. Hold. Relax.
9. With arms straight by your side, palms down, bend the fingers up and back toward the arm, bending at the wrist. Hold. Relax.
10. Bend the elbows and repeat step 9, bending the hands back toward the shoulders. Hold. Relax.
11. Make a tight fist of your hands, bring the arms out to the sides and move the arms up perpendicular to the floor. Move very slowly, resisting the movement all the while to make the pectoral muscles of the bust stand out.
12. Pull the shoulderblades of the back together. Hold. Relax.
13. Pull the shoulders up beside the ears. Hold. Relax.
14. Pull down the corners of the mouth. Hold. Relax.
15. Bring the tongue to the back of the roof of the mouth. Hold. Relax.
16. Purse your lips, wrinkle the nose and squeeze the eyes tightly shut. Hold. Relax.
17. Smile with the lips closed and stretch the face. Hold. Relax.

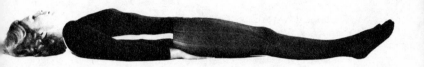

(Figure 111)

18. Yawn very slowly, resisting the movement.
19. Press the back of the head against the floor. Hold. Relax.
20. Frown, moving the scalp forward. Hold. Relax.
21. Go through the eye exercises.
22. Pull your head under and against the shoulders without moving anything else.
23. Relax, melting into the floor, for up to 10 minutes. (Figure 111)

III. *Dos and Don'ts:*

DO hold each holding position for at least 5 seconds.
DO relax after each holding position, by flopping back into place after each flexing position.
DO NOT worry or think of unpleasant things as you relax at the end of the Sponge. Rather keep your thoughts to a minimum, on pleasant things, and dispassionately watch them wander past without trying to become involved.

The Sponge is called the Dead Man's Pose or Corpse in the Sanskrit language. Really, it is a deep relaxation pose where your body has a chance to assimilate what it has learned, at its leisure. Seldom do we take the time simply to relax. We may read, watch T.V. or sleep. Just because we lie down does not at all mean we are relaxing our deep-seated neuro-muscular tensions. The body has to relearn how to do that. After some weeks of the deliberate Sponge technique you will find that you can relax without going through all the steps.

SPREAD LEG STRETCH

I.   *Benefits:*

The Spread Leg Stretch —
- stretches, firms and makes *shapely* the hamstring muscles of the *legs.*
- removes *tension* of *whole body.*
- beneficial to entire *pelvic area* (circulation).
- relieves pains of *sciatica.*
- especially beneficial to women: regulates *menstruation* and stimulates proper function of ovaries.
- firms and reduces weight in the *thighs.*
- limbers up and makes the *spine* flexible.

II. *Technique:*

1. Sit on the floor, legs outstretched and as far apart as possible. (Figure 112)
2. Place your hands on your legs and slowly slide them down toward the toes. Keep the legs straight.
3. Bending forward from the waist, in a curling motion, bring your hands as far as they can go, then grasp that part of the leg you can comfortably reach. (Figure 113)
4. Let your head hang down and bend the elbows to give a good forward stretch. Hold for 10 - 30 seconds. Relax, slowly return. (Figure 114 — Advanced Pose)

5. Repeat twice more.

III. *Dos and Don'ts:*

DO sit well back on your pelvis, not on your tailbone.
DO NOT bend your knees, you will nullify many of the benefits.
DO NOT jerk or bounce.

In the advanced form of this pose, you will be able to lower your head to the floor, which will give you the added benefit of improved circulation to the head. It is a particularly beneficial pose for ladies and recommended for daily use.

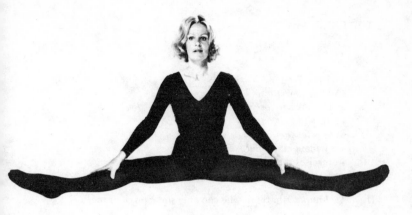

(Figure 112)

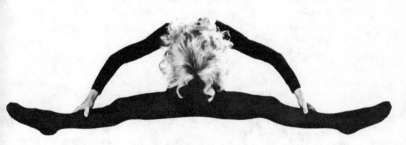

(Figure 113)

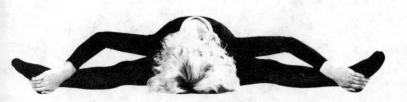

(Figure 114)

TOE EXERCISE

I. *Benefits:*

The Toe Exercise ——
- strengthens *toes*.
- prevents *varicose veins*.
- aids *elimination*.
- eases *tension*.
- is beneficial for *flat feet*.
- exercises the *knee joint*.

II. *Technique:* for those who can only squat on their toes:

1. Squat, knees apart, arms hanging straight forward between the knees for better balance. (Figure 115)
2. Balance on the toes and slowly attempt to lower the heels to the floor. Go as far as you can and then hold for 5 - 20 seconds.
3. Come up on the toes again slowly and relax by sitting down if necessary.
4. Repeat 3 times.
5. Gradually bring knees closer together.

III. *Technique:* for those who can comfortably squat on their heels:

1. Squat, knees apart, arms hanging straight forward between the knees. (Figure 116)
2. Slowly rise up on the toes and balance there for 5 - 20 seconds.
3. Come slowly back down onto the heels.
4. Repeat three times.
5. Gradually bring knees closer together.

IV. *Dos and Don'ts:*

DO put emphasis on whatever comes not very easily. If you find it easy to balance on your toes, then practice bringing the heels down and vice-versa.

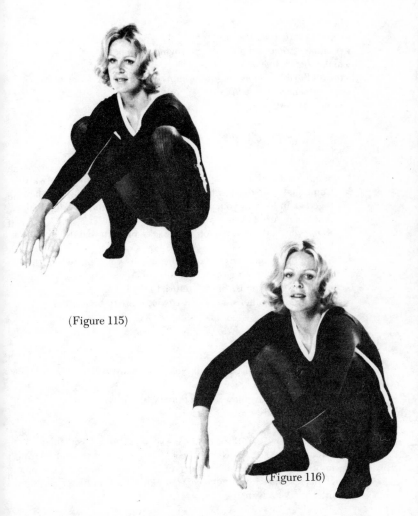

(Figure 115)

(Figure 116)

The Toe Exercise strengthens not only the toes but is beneficial to the whole foot and the legs. It is one of those "many-benefits-combined-in-one" exercises, even though it seems to be more obscure.

TOE TWIST

I.   *Benefits:*

The Toe Twist ——
- reduces *waistline.*
- promotes *grace* and poise by improving *balance.*
- makes *legs shapely.*
- makes flexible and *massages the spine* through cork-screw twist.
- strengthens *feet* and *ankles.*
- improves *posture.*

II.   *Technique:*

1.   Stand erect with your feet together, toes slightly pointed outward.
2.   Come slowly up on your toes, at the same time bringing both hands together in front of you, arms straight, thumbs interlocking, palms down. (Figure 117)
3.   Keep your eyes riveted on the backs of your hands for better balance.
4.   Slowly bring the arms as far to the side as you can, twisting from the waist and keeping the toes firmly dug in.
5.   Hold 10 - 20 seconds. Slowly return to the front.
6.   Repeat on the other side. Repeat twice more to both sides.

III. *Dos and Don'ts:*

DO NOT become distracted if you lose your balance. Simply try again.
DO NOT in any way allow your toes to swivel as you twist.
DO keep your body straight, chest out.

The Toe Twist works on almost every portion of your body, but most important perhaps is the effect it has on your general bearing. By improving your balance, you gain confidence in your movement which makes for poise and grace. Your clothes will fit better and show to much greater advantage.

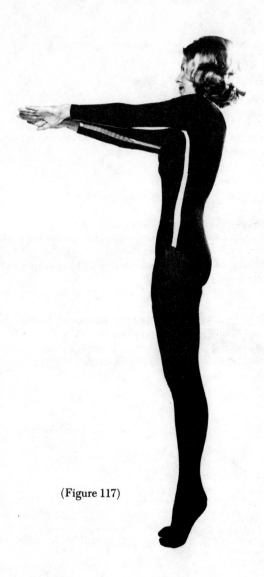

(Figure 117)

TREE (Stork)

I.   *Benefits:*

The Tree —
- improves *circulation* in *lower extremities.*
- promotes *poise* and *grace* through improving *balance.*
- teaches proper posture since body must be perfectly aligned to keep balance.
- tones the *leg muscles.*

II. *Technique:*

1.   Stand with your feet together, arms by your side.
2.   Bend the right leg and prop the sole of the foot against the left thigh.
3.   Bring the heel as close to the perineum as possible and rest the foot there, pointing the knee to the side. (Figure 119)
4.   Bring the palms together and raise the hands straight over the head. (Figure 120)
5.   Hold as long as balance permits and breathe deeply.
6.   Lower the leg and hands slowly and relax.
7.   Repeat with the left leg.
8.   Repeat twice more on both sides.

III. *Dos and Don'ts:*

DO prop your foot slightly to the front of the thigh for better support. It has a tendency to slide if too far back.

DO practice your balancing first, if necessary, by keeping the arms out to the sides for better balance.

DO NOT come out of the pose suddenly.

Balance must be kept conditioned just as much as muscle-tone, but it is more quickly regained with practice. Balance whenever possible, perhaps while conversing on the phone.

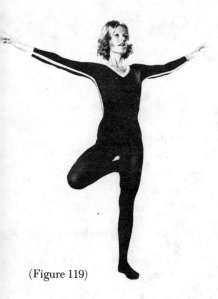

(Figure 119)

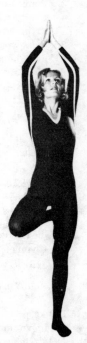

(Figure 120)

TRIANGLE POSTURE

I. *Benefits:*

The Triangle Posture ——
- relieves *back-ache*.
- develops *chest*.
- relieves *menstrual problems*.
- tones *hip, thigh* and *leg muscles*.
- massages and stimulates *abdominal organs*.
- slims the *waist* in the variation.

II. *Technique:*

1. Stand with the feet 3 feet apart.
2. Bring your arms out straight at the sides, parallel to the floor. (Figure 121)
3. Point your right foot 90°, the left foot slightly to the right.
4. Bend your body to the right, bringing the hand as close as possible to the outside of the right foot.
5. Bring your left arm up so that it is in a straight line with the right arm. Look up at the left hand. (Figure 122)
6. Hold 10 - 30 seconds, breathing normally.
7. Come up slowly.
8. Repeat on the other side.
9. Repeat twice more on each side.

Variation:

1. Do steps 1 - 3 as above.
2. With arms out-stretched, twist your body to the right and bring the left arm as close as possible to the outside of the right foot.
3. Bring your right arm up in back so that it is in a straight line with the left one. Look up at the right hand. (Figure 123)
4. Complete steps 6, 7, 8, and 9 as above.

III. *Dos and Don'ts:*

DO keep both your knees absolutely straight throughout. It is not so important how far you go as that you do it properly.
DO stretch your shoulders as you hold.

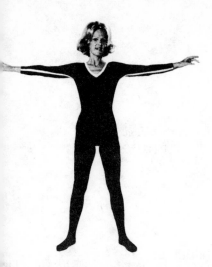

(Figure 121)

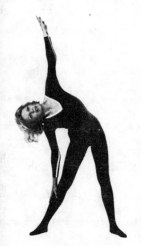

(Figure 122)

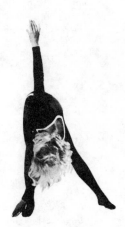

(Figure 123)

The Triangle Postures are very reminiscent of calisthenics with the tremendous difference of the tension-dissolving holding action. Try them both and see the difference.

TWIST

I. *Benefits:*

    The Twist —
    • firms and reduces *waist*.
    • makes the *hipjoint* flexible.
    • massages *abdominal organs* to aid digestion.
    • makes *spine* limber which has therapeutic effect on *nervous system*
    • realigns *vertebrae* and relieves *tension*.
    • tones *muscles* and *firms figure*.

II. *Technique:*

    1. Sit on the floor, legs outstretched.
    2. Spread your legs and bring the *right foot* against the *left thigh.*
        Press the side of the right knee against the floor. (Figure 124)
    3. Bend your left knee and, leaving it sticking up in the air, bring the
        left foot over the *right knee*. (Figure 125)
    4. Set the sole of the *left foot* squarely on the floor. The further back
        you can bring the foot, the better.
    5. Using both hands for support, shift your weight well forward onto
        the pelvis, to prevent tipping.
    6. With the *left hand* behind you on the floor for support, raise your
        right arm and bring it between your chest and the left knee. (Fig-
        ure 126)
    7. Twist your body so that you *right shoulder* is resting against the
        left knee.
    8. Now make a fist of your *right hand* and move your *right arm* poker
        straight over the *right knee* that is lying on the floor.
    9. Attempt to get hold of the toes of the left foot. As a beginner, that
        is nearly impossible, so it is perfectly alright to grasp the right
        knee. (Figure 127)
    10. Levering yourself against the *left leg* with the *right arm*, now twist
        to the left.
    11. Bend your left arm and bring the back of the hand against the
        small of the back.
    12. Turn your head to the left and look as far left as you can. (Figure
        128)
    13. Hold this position for 10 - 30 seconds.
    14. Slowly unwind.
    15. Repeat on the other side.

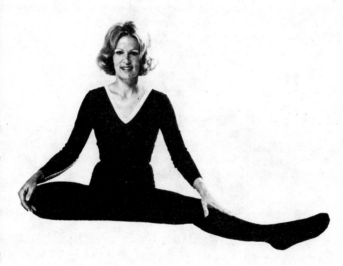

(Figure 124)

II. *Dos and Don'ts:*

DO sit well forward on your pelvis.
DO NOT bend your arm as you draw it across the knee.
DO swivel your shoulder or upper arm against the knee to permit you
    to bring your arm around further.

    The Twist seems like an almost impossible position to assume at
first. A picture here is worth a 1,000 words. Once you have the idea,
however, the Twist will become a most satisfying exercise because it
stretches most muscles of the body. The spiral twist that the spine is
getting is most beneficial too.

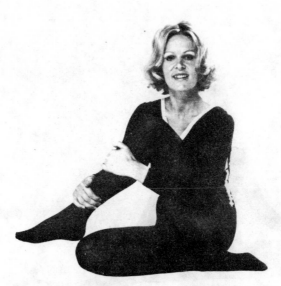

(Figure 125)

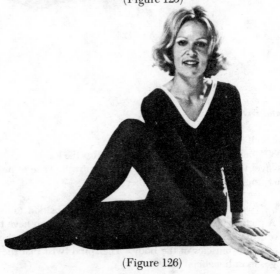

(Figure 126)

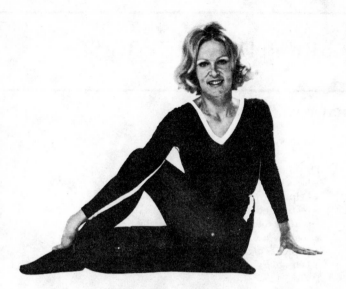

(Figure 127)

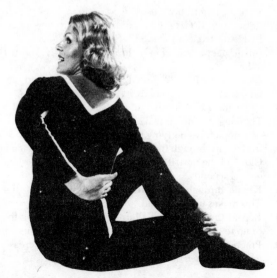

(Figure 128)

BREATHING EXERCISES

ALTERNATE NOSTRIL BREATH

I.   *Benefits:*

The Alternate Nostril Breath ——
- has a marvellously calming effect on the *nervous system*.
- helps to overcome *insomnia*.
- *relaxes* and *refreshes* the body.
- purifies the *bloodstream* and aerates the *lungs*.
- soothes *headaches*.
- improves *digestion* and *appetite*.
- helps to free the mind of *anxiety* and *depression*.

II.   *Technique:*

1.   Sit in a comfortably cross-legged position, back straight.
2.   Raise your RIGHT hand and place your ringfinger against yo
      LEFT nostril, closing it off. (Figure 129)
3.   Inhale deeply and slowly through the RIGHT nostril to the cou
      of four.
4.   Close off the RIGHT nostril with your thumb and retain the brea
      for a count of 1 - 4 seconds.   (Figure 129a)
5.   Open the LEFT nostril and exhale to the count of 4 - 8 secon
      The longer you can make the exhalation, the better. Concentra
      on completely emptying the lungs.
6.   Breathe in through that same LEFT nostril to the count of 4.
7.   Close off the nostril with the ringfinger again and hold to the cou
      of 1 - 4 seconds.
8.   Exhale through the RIGHT nostril to the count of 4 - 8 secon
      This makes up one round.
9.   Repeat these rounds of alternate nostril breathing five more tim
      or up to ten minutes if you are concerned about insomnia.
10.   Practice a ratio of 4:4:8, if at all possible. Increase this to 8:4
      eventually, then 8:8:8, after some months.

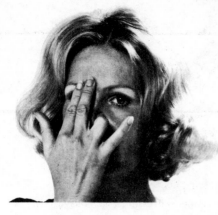

(Figure 129)

(Figure 129a)

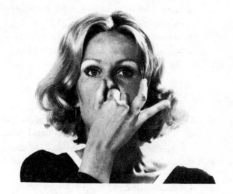

II. *Dos and Don'ts:*

DO NOT push yourself with the holding position or by increasing the ratio until you are comfortable doing so.

DO make the breathing rhythmic, smooth and slow. You can work on making it inaudible eventually.

DO practice the Alternate Nostril Breath whenever you need calming -- if you are nervous, upset or irritable.

I cannot over-emphasize the importance of this particular breath. The body and mind are closely inter-related and one influences the other to a much greater extent than medicine admitted to for many years. As an all-round "soother" the Alternate Nostril Breath is incomparable.

THE CLEANSING BREATH

I. *Benefits:*

The Cleansing Breath ——
- clears *lungs, sinuses* and nasal passages.
- relieves *colds*.
- tones the *nervous system*.
- strengthens the *lungs, thorax* and *abdomen*.
- purifies the *bloodstream* and clears the *head*.
- aids *digestion*.
- stimulates the *liver, spleen* and *pancreas*.

II. *Technique:*

1. Sit in a comfortably cross-legged position or a chair, back straight.
2. Inhale deeply, pushing the abdomen out, and taking in as much a
    as possible in the space of 1 second. (Figure 130)
3. Whack your abdomen in forcefully to expel the air through th
    nostrils. The sensation should be one of having been punched i
    the stomach. (Figure 131)
4. Inhale again by pushing the abdomen out and letting the air rus
    back into the vacuum created by the exhalation.
5. The whole process, inhalation and exhalation, should take no
    much more than 1½ seconds. Both should be forceful and will b
    quite audible.
6. Repeat ten times, follow with a complete breath and repeat te
    times more.

III. *Dos and Don'ts:*

DO push the abdomen out as far as you can as you inhale.
DO NOT exhale consciously, but let the action of the abdomen do
    for you.

The Cleansing Breath is a cross between the Bellows Breath whic
is more difficult and the Dynamic Cleansing Breath. It has a ma
vellous effect of clearing the cobwebs out of your mind and is recon
mended before any task in which you need energy and ment
alertness.

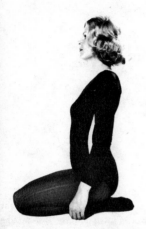

(Figure 130)

(Figure 131)

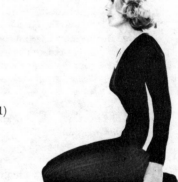

COMPLETE BREATH

I. *Benefits:*

The Complete Breath ——
- recharges *energy*.
- purifies the *bloodstream* and enriches it.
- develops *chest* and *diaphragm*.
- strengthens *lungs, thorax* and *abdomen*.
- increases resistance to *colds*.
- calms the *nervous system*.
- aids *digestion*.
- clears up *phlegm*.
- helps to lift *depression*.

II. *Technique:*

1. Sit in a comfortably cross-legged position or in a chair.
2. Straighten your back, which will straighten your thorax for easie breathing.
3. Inhale *slowly* through the nose, breathing deeply, consciously.
4. Take five seconds to fill the lower part of the lungs, by expandin the ribs and pushing the abdomen out. (Figure 132)
5. Concentrate on filling the top of the lungs for the next five seconds This will expand the chest and tighten the abdomen slightly.
6. Hold the breath for 1 - 5 seconds.
7. Exhale slowly until you have emptied the lungs. (Figure 133)
8. Repeat 4 - 5 times more.

III. *Dos and Don'ts:*

DO establish a rhythmic rise and fall of your abdomen, to promote regular breathing.

DO attempt to breathe inaudibly after you have gotten the knack o deep breathing.

DO NOT slump. For maximum efficiency the thorax must be straight

DO concentrate on your breathing alone, with your eyes closed, if you wish. It serves to do the technique better but it is also a prepar ation for meditation.

DO push your abdomen out as you breathe in and pull the abdomen i as you breathe out.

DO give an extra snort as you exhale to rid yourself of stale waste matter in the bottom of the lungs.

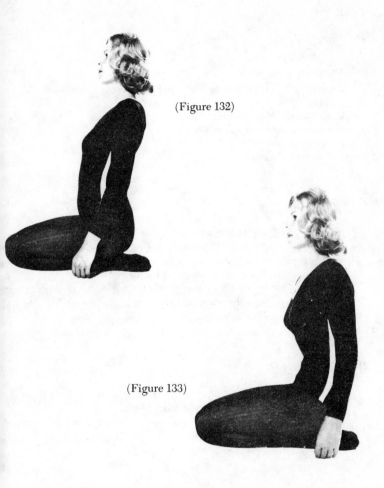

(Figure 132)

(Figure 133)

Oxygen is our most important food and the customary shallow breathing of most people can be compared to the hasty swallowing of food: both cause immeasurable health-problems. If you regularly breathe deeply you can revitalize yourself and rid yourself of the chronic fatigue so common to housewives; you can improve your mental outlook, your digestion and your general health by resisting respiratory ailments.

COOLING BREATH

I. *Benefits:*

The Cooling Breath —
- has a cooling effect on the body, and is particularly recommended for *fever*
- purifies the *bloodstream.*
- prevents *respiratory ailments.*
- aids *digestion.*
- *decreases* the *appetite.*

II. *Technique:*

1. Sit in a comfortably cross-legged position, back straight.
2. Form your tongue into a trough and let it protude slightly from the lips. (Figure 134)
3. Inhale air through this trough with a hissing sound.
4. Hold your breath for 1 - 5 seconds.
5. Exhale through the nostrils.
6. Repeat 5 more times.

III. *Dos and Don'ts:*

DO encourage your child to practice this breath before he is ill, so that he is familiar with it when he has a fever.

DO NOT inhale too forcefully, but make it a steady, slow pull, expanding the chest and abdomen.

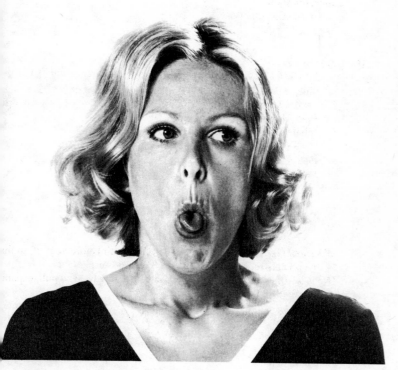

(Figure 134)

PROBLEMS

EXERCISES FOR SPECIFIC AREAS

1. *ABDOMEN:*
   Pump, Abdominal Lift, Sit-Up, Rock n' Rolls, Plough, Bow, Alternate Leg Stretch, Locust (Boat), Chest Expander, Cross Beam, Forward Bend Sitting, Mountain, Leg-Over

2. *ARMS and WRISTS:*
   Arm Lift, Cobra-On-Toes, Crow, Arm and Leg Stretch, Posture Clasp, Chest Expander, Fountain, Bow, Cat Stretch

3. *ANKLES:*
   Ankle Bends, Triangle Postures, Sitting Warrior, Cobra-On-Toes, Frog, Knee and Thigh Stretch, Dog Stretch (advanced), Cross Beam

4. *BACK and SPINE:*
   Forward Bend, Alternate Leg Stretch, Twist, Cat Stretch, Plough, Bow, Cobra, Boat, Leg-Over, Chest Expander, Cross Beam, Camel, Pendulum, Pump

5. *BUST and CHEST:*
   Chest Expander, Arms-To-Wall, Posture Clasp, Cobra, Bow, Fish, Pelvic Stretch, Arm and Leg Stretch, Triangle Postures

6. *BUTTOCKS:*
   Locust, Cobra, Pelvic Stretch, Shoulderstand, Plough, Bow, Alternate Leg Stretch, Pump, Sit-Up

7. *CIRCULATION:*
   Shoulderstand, Headstand Walk-Up, Pump, Symbol of Yoga, Plough, Chest Expander, Cobra, Curling Leaf, Pendulum, Mountain, Tree

8. *EYES:*
   Eye Exercises, Lion, Shoulderstand, Headstand Walk-Up, Neck Rolls

9. *FACE:*
    Lion, Beauty Breath or Symbol Of Yoga, Shoulderstand, Plough, Forward Bend Standing

10. *FEET:*
    Japanese Sitting Position, Perfect Posture, Pelvic Stretch, Frog, Sitting Warrior, Toe Twist

12. *KNEES:*
    Alternate Leg Stretch, Knee and Thigh Stretch, Sitting Warrior, Frog, Twist, Toe Exercise

13. *HIPS:*
    Locust (Boat), Half Locust, Ankle To Forehead Stretch, Triangle Posture, Bow, Fountain, Twist (hip-joint)

14. *LEGS:*
    Toe Twist, Sitting Warrior, Shoulderstand, Frog, Dog Stretch (advanced), Tree, Stork, Arm and Leg Stretch, Perfect Posture, Alternate Leg Stretch, Bow, Forward Bend Sitting, Curling Leaf

15. *NECK and CHIN:*
    Neck Rolls, Chest Expander, Fish, Cobra, Plough, Cat Stretch

16. *POSTURE and SHOULDERS:*
    Posture Clasp, Blade, Chest Expander, Tree, Stork, Arm and Leg Stretch, Bow, Pelvic Stretch, Pendulum, Cobra, Plough, Arm Lift, Camel

17. *THIGHS:*
    Knee and Thigh Stretch, Spread Leg Stretch, Alternate Leg Stretch, Triangle Posture, Perfect Posture, Pelvic Stretch, Arm and Leg Stretch, Cross Beam

18. *TOES:*
    Toe Balance, Pelvic Stretch, Toe Twist

19. *TENSION:*
>Neck Rolls, Lion, Cobra, Shoulderstand, Fish, Chest Expander, Rock n' Rolls, Forward Bend (Knee and Thigh), Alternate Leg Stretch, Eye Exercises, Curling Leaf, Sponge

20. *WAIST and MIDRIFF:*
>Twist, Triangle Posture (Side Bend), Toe Twist, Leg-Over, Fountain, Abdominal Lift, Pump

EXERCISES FOR SPECIFIC HEALTH PROBLEMS

1. *ANEMIA*
   Shoulderstand, Both Forward Bends, Sponge (10 - 15 mins.), Complete Breath

2. *ARTHRITIS* (of the Back):
   Triangle Posture, Mountain, Curling Leaf, Twist, Forward Bend Standing, Shoulderstand, Cobra, Locust

3. *ASTHMA:*
   Fish, Shoulderstand, Mountain, Locust, Alternate Leg Stretch, Both Forward Bends, Cobra

4. *BURSITIS:*
   Blade, Pendulum, Chest Expander, Posture Clasp

5. *BACKACHE:*
   All Standing Poses, Shoulderstand, Leg-Over, Symbol Of Yoga (Maha Mudra), Alternate Leg Stretch

6. *HIGH BLOOD PRESSURE:*
   Plough, Alternate Leg Stretch, Forward Bend Sitting, Symbol Of Yoga, Alternate Nostril Breathing, Sponge

7. *BREATHLESSNESS:*
   Both Forward Bends, Plough, Shoulderstand, Mountain, All Breathing Exercises, Sponge

8. *COLD:*
   Shoulderstand, Both Forward Bends, Complete Breath

9. *CONSTIPATION:*
   Abdominal Lift, Both Forward Bends, Twist, Plough, Triangle Postures, Fish, Alternate Leg Stretch, Shoulderstand, Toe Exercises

10. *DIABETES:*

Symbol Of Yoga, Shoulderstand, Twist, Alternate Leg Stretch, Plough, Fish, Mountain, Locust, Forward Bend Sitting

11. *DISPLACED DISC:*

Cat Stretch, Forward Bend Sitting, Locust (Boat), All Standing Postures, Bow, Camel, Cobra, Fish, Shoulderstand

12. *FATIGUE:*

Shoulderstand, Headstand Walk-Up, Plough, Chest Expander, Both Forward Bends, Twist, Curling Leaf, Alternate Nostril Breathing Without Retention, Complete Breath, Ankle Bends

13. *FLAT FEET:*

Shoulderstand, Sitting and Reclining Warrior, Frog, Knee and Thigh Stretch

14. *GALL BLADDER:*

Triangle Postures, Both Forward Bends, Shoulderstand, Alternate Leg Stretch, Twist, Locust

15. *HEADACHE:*

Headstand Walk-Up For Protracted Time, Shoulderstand (For 3 mins. or more), Plough, Forward Bends, Alternate Nostril Breathing Without Retention, Eye Exercises, Neck Rolls

16. *HEART TROUBLE:*

Breathing Exercises; Complete and Alternate Nostril Without Retention, Sponge

17. *HEELS* (Calcaneal spurs or pain):

Shoulderstand, *Sitting Warrior,* Triangle (formed by legs on arms on floor, pressing the heels toward the floor), Frog, Knee and Thigh Stretch

18. *INDIGESTION:*

Shoulderstand, Twist, Cobra, Bow, Locust, Symbol Of Yoga, Plough, Mountain, Pump

19. *INSOMNIA:*

Shoulderstand, Cobra, Forward Bend Sitting, Mountain, Bellows Breath, Plough, Alternate Nostril Breath, Neck Rolls

20. *KIDNEYS:*
    Shoulderstand, Standing Poses, Cobra-On-Toes, Locust (Boat), Bow, Alternate Leg Stretch, Forward Bend Sitting, Knee and Thigh Stretch, Spread Leg Stretch, Leg-Over, Twist, Plough

21. *LUMBAGO:*
    Plough, Locust, Bow, Cobra, Sponge

22. *MENSTRUAL DISORDERS and OVARIES:*
    Both Forward Bends, Dog Stretch (advanced), Symbol Of Yoga, Mountain, Fish, Sitting and Reclining Warrior, Spread Leg Stretch, Knee and Thigh Stretch, Shoulderstand, Cobra, Cat Stretch, Triangle Postures

23. *OBESITY* (weight control):
    Plough, Triangle Postures, Cobra, Both Forward Bends, Locust, Twist, Shoulderstand

24. *PALPITATIONS:*
    Shoulderstand, Plough, Both Forward Bends, Dog Stretch (advanced), Sitting Warrior, Complete Breath, Alternate Nostril Breath Without Retention at the Beginning, Sponge

25. *PILES:*
    Fish, Plough, Shoulderstand, Leg-Over, Locust (Boat), Bow

26. *PROSTATES:*
    Leg-Over, Forward Bend Standing, Locust (Boat), Bow, Dog Stretch (advanced), Staff (advanced), Alternate Leg Stretch, Sitting and Reclining Warrior, Knee and Thigh Stretch, Lotus

27. *RHEUMATISM:*
    Twist, Forward Bend Sitting, Plough, Mountain, Boat, Alternate Leg Stretch, Shoulderstand

28. *SCIATICA.*
    Leg-Over, Alternate Leg Stretch, Both Forward Bends, Shoulderstand, Knee and Thigh Stretch, Boat, Bow, Cobra, Spread Leg Stretch

29. *SEXUAL DEBILITY:*
    Shoulderstand, Abdominal Lift, Symbol Of Yoga

30. *URINE* (dribbling):
> Shoulderstand, Sitting and Reclining (advanced) Warrior, Fish, Trunk Sealer (advanced), Knee and Thigh Stretch, Abdominal Lift, Perfect Postures

31. *VARICOSE VEINS:*
> Shoulderstand, Sitting and Reclining (advanced) Warrior, Frog, Curling Leaf

EXERCISE
SCHEDULES

1. THE GROUP OF TWELVE (MOST IMPORTANT)

1. Rockn' Rolls
2. Headstand Attempt
3. Shoulderstand
4. Pelvic Stretch
5. Plough
6. Cobra
7. Forward Bend Standing
8. Fish
9. Twist
10. Bow
11. Alternate Leg Stretch
12. Lion

Of the over 70 exercises we practice on the T.V.-show there are many I consider as important as the ones above. However, for a program which exercises almost all organs and muscles of the body, this is the best combination. You can extend the time it takes you to work through these exercises according to your preference or ability. It can easily be a fifteen minute program. You would do each exercise for 5 seconds, relax and repeat it as often as you can in one minute.

If you are quite advanced, you can hold each exercise for 30 - 60 seconds and only do it once. But if you are less ambitious, you can make this an hour-long, or longer program taking time out for resting between exercises.

2. A FIFTEEN MINUTE PROGRAM

1. Headstand Attempt
2. Shoulderstand
3. Cobra
4. Forward Bend Sitting
5. Pelvic Stretch

If you only have a little time, practice at least these exercises, daily. Substitute any exercise that you particularly need, i.e. the Pump for a flabby abdomen, or the Abdominal Lift for constipation.

3. AN EXERCISE PROGRAM FOR SLIMMING

1. Fountain
2. Shoulderstand
3. Bow
4. Plough
5. Fish
6. Abdominal Lift
7. Pump
8. Twist

Include in this list any exercise you know to be beneficial for your particular fatty area. If you are unsure, please check the list at the back of the book called "EXERCISES FOR SPECIFIC AREAS".

4. EXERCISES FOR THE OFFICE

1. Chest Expander
2. Alternate Nostril Breathing
3. Twist in a Chair
4. Stork
5. Forward Bend Standing
6. Neck Rolls
7. Posture Clasp

Much better than any coffee-break is time-out for energy-producing exercises. In Russia, workers now go through a half-hour exercise program instead of the coffee-break and have been found to be considerably more productive. Get your fellow-workers to exercise with you -- it will keep them from laughing at you, in their ignorance.

5. EXERCISES FOR EXPECTANT MOTHERS

1. Mountain
2. Complete Breath With Suspension
3. Toe Balance (squat)
4. Cat Stretch (first two movements)
5. Tree (with chair for support, if necessary)
6. Knee and Thigh Stretch
7. Hands-to-Wall

It is quite safe to exercise for the first three months of the pregnancy if you have no record of miscarriage. However, check with your doctor first. Of greatest importance is the squatting position, followed by the back-strengthening Cat Stretch.

6. YOGA FOR CHILDREN

1. Cat Stretch
2. Complete Breath
3. Stork - Balance - Hopping
4. Plough - Backward Roll
5. Shoulderstand
6. Cobra
7. Wheel
8. Forward Bend - Tree
9. Lion
10. Sponge - Rag Doll

Children also love Yoga and are enthusiastic, faithful students. But since their muscles must be in constant movement for better development, a modified version of Hatha Yoga is advised. For instance, let them pretend to be a cat or a lion, with all the accompanying noises. In the Complete Breath put a rubber duck or boat on their abdomen, and have them pretend it is floating in the rising and falling waves of their tummy. The Stork need not be immobile but can, after a while, hop around on one foot, flapping its wings. Have the children close their eyes to test their balance. The Plough can develop into a backward roll by bringing the hands near the shoulders, pointing the fingers toward the body and giving a little push. If they roll to the side, they are not exerting equal pressure on both hands. The Wheel can be practiced by standing some distance away from the wall, back towards it, and crawling down backwards on the wall. The Forward Bend can easily represent a tree swaying in a stronger and stronger breeze till finally he snaps in two. And the Sponge is a limp rag doll. Teach them, the pleasure will be yours shared.

7. A SPLIT SCHEDULE

MORNING:

1. Chest Expander
2. Dynamic Cleansing Breath
3. Forward Bend Standing
4. Pelvic Stretch
5. Triangle Posture
6. Knee and Thigh Stretch
7. Toe Twist
8. Arm and Leg Stretch
9. Eye Exercises

EVENING:

1. Pump
2. Yoga Mudra
3. Shoulderstand
4. Lion
5. Twist
6. Trunk Sealer
7. Bow
8. Plough
9. Cobra
10. Neck Rolls
11. Alternate Nostril Breathing
12. Sponge

8. YOGA FOR WOULD-BE NON-SMOKERS

For trying to quit smoking, one of the best techniques is to accustom your system once again to a phenomenon called "fresh air". This is best accomplished by performing as often as possible the following breathing exercises:

1. Dynamic Cleansing Breath
2. Complete Breath
3. The Alternate Nostril Breath

Perform the first two before and after each exercise session, any time you are in fresh air and any time you feel the urge to smoke. The Alternate Nostril Breath is best done at bedtime. If you have been a heavy smoker there will be a tendency to hyperventilate -- that is, to feel slightly dizzy or overcome by the unaccustomed flood of oxygen. There is no need for alarm and the sensation will pass as your body adjusts to the new, healthful, life-prolonging breathing habits.

IMPULSE YOGA

What is Impulse Yoga? Officially, it doesn't exist. It's a term I have coined in the effort to communicate with my "invisible" viewers. It's Self-Awareness; it's Yoga incorporated into your day; it's being tuned in to your own B-O-D-Y channel.

What the body has to tell you is very important. The impulses it sends out are sent for a reason. In Arabia, for example, where it is impolite NOT to burp, there is a much lower incidence of digestive problems. Don't let the taboos of our society force you into poor health. Get others involved in a good stretch, arch, or flexing, too. Tell them that it is detensionizing. Learn to speak your own body language again. Babies know how. We adults have become experts in the vice of suppression — to the detriment of body and mind. LISTEN inward and then do what you're told! There is a reason for your impulse: better health.

1. STRETCH — *whenever* or *wherever* your body feels kinked or cramped. Copy the cat. Stretching is tranquilizing.
2. GRUNT or GROAN — whenever you stretch. Let yourself go, totally. It is marvellously relaxing to follow all body impulses — to be off one's guard, for once!
3. YAWN — don't ever suppress it. Yawning is the body's demand for oxygen NOW. It doesn't mean you're bored, at all. It simply means that the room is stuffy. Yawning wakes up the brain cells, makes you alert. So, if you're trying to sleep, don't yawn.
4. ARCH and BEND — how often one feels like bending back in a chair, after being hunched over a task for hours. How often one would like to collapse in half, like a ragdoll. Do it!
5. FLEX and CONTRACT — toes, hamstrings, fingers, whatever. If that is what your body wants to do, let it. Contract, the better to relax afterward.
6. MASSAGE or SCRATCH — be good to yourself, give yourself a massage or pummel that slipped hip. But do it, or have it done, when the body asks for it. Remember, it has a reason for that particular timing.
7. SNEEZE — try not to suppress it, but please cover your mouth and nose. Sneezing has a marvellous cleansing effect, helping to rid the nose of irritating matter.
8. BURPS — may be caused by food allergy, ulcers, gas-producing food combinations or other reasons. Check with your doctor. Burp discreetly, but do not suppress.

9. VOID — whenever possible, as soon as the urge appears. Too full bladders can eventually lead to various health problems and constipation may actually permit reabsorption of toxins into the body. You will find that you become more alert mentally.

10. LISTEN TO YOUR BODY IMPULSES — all the time.

TRIGGER YOGA

Just as the word *yoga* has nothing to do with yogurt or yo-yos, so the word *trigger* does not refer to a horse or the part of a pistol. Instead, it means that the repetitive stimuli we are all exposed to every day should automatically trigger the thought: "Aha, this is the perfect time for me to practise my . . . (such and such) yoga exercise." For instance, every time you come to a red light, (as driver or passenger) it should remind you that this is the time to work on your pectorals, to offset wrinkles or to relieve a sore throat. In other words, press your hands against the steering wheel or do the LION! That exercise will even work off aggressive feelings caused by the stresses of city driving.

Can you see the possibilities? You can do yoga, ANYTIME, ANYWHERE – without really trying! People often ask me how many hours of yoga I do a day. The answer is: none! I do it ALL DAY LONG.

I am sure that you can add your own TRIGGER YOGA ideas to the list. If you do, please let me in on the secret. I'd love to do more yoga! ANYTIME!

1. Waking up in the Morning:
    SIDE STRETCH in bed, keeping shoulders steady. Try to stretch each hand in turn, as though to reach the foot.

2. Brushing Teeth:
    ALTERNATE LEG STRETCH VARIATION: Bring one foot up on toilet lid, windowsill or even sink, bend into extended leg and brush. Change sides. (Also see p. 20.)

3. Red Light:
    HANDS-TO-WALL (Steering Wheel): Slowly bend elbows, resisting the movement, 'til the forehead touches wheel. Return slowly, resisting. (More on p. 60.)

4. Brushing Hair:
    FORWARD BEND STANDING, keeping knees straight, hand loose and brush hair. With each brushstroke try to go a little further down. (More on p. 56.)

5. On the Phone:
    BALANCING POSES: Do the Tree Stand on one leg, slowly pulling the other one along the inside of the first. Hold as long as you can. If necessary, lean with hip lightly against counter. (See page 108.)

6. In the Kitchen:
   SQUAT whenever you peel anything. TOE TWIST every time you get something out of the cupboard. Stand with your back to the counter, come lightly up on toes, twist to reach. (See p. 104 for more.)

7. Picking anything up:
   ABDOMINAL LIFT: Bend forward while exhaling, relax and let your abdomen get pulled in all by itself. Hold, inhale, straighten, and relax. Does wonders for the muscles and the digestion! (Detailed instructions page 18.)

8. At the Desk:
   CHEST EXPANDER SITTING: Sit at the edge of your chair with legs apart, clasp your hands behind your back, exhale and bend forward, pushing the hands as high up in the air as you can. (See p. 38 for detailed description.)

9. In the Car, Plane or Bus:
   ISOMETRIC EXERCISES: Press the head against the back of the seat, hold; put hands on knees, press hard as though to stand up; tense individual muscles, then relax them; lift shoulders up, back, forward, rotate; roll neck slowly around.

10. At a Dinner Party:
    ASWINI MUDRA: Arrange to be seated opposite your date, take off your shoes and put your feet on his lap; or pinch the buttocks together, hold, relax. Repeat many times.

11. In Front of the TV:
    SIT-UPS: Sit with the knees drawn up just enough to let the whole sole of the foot touch. Bring arms behind head and very slowly lie down. (Beginners can hook feet under the couch, and use one elbow for support.) (See page 98.)

    BACK BENDS such as the ROCKING BOW: Lie on your tummy, grab ankles (with hands or the aid of scarves), exhale, pull the ankles away from the hands, head up. Breathe fairly deeply, so that your breath rocks you. Relax, repeat.

    ROCKN' ROLLS (See page 90.)

    SPREAD LEG STRETCH SITTING: Spread your legs as wide as you comfortably can, bend forward from the waist, place bent elbows on the floor, wrists together, and rest your head in your cupped hands. Hold indefinitely. (See page 102.)

    LEG-OVER (see page 70): Position yourself so that the crossing leg is hooked against something and your face is in the direction of the T.V. Hold a long time.

12. Anytime, Anywhere:
    Take your pick from the above or invent your own.

INDEX